HOMEOPATHIC REMEDIES FOR DOGS

Geoffrey Llewellyn

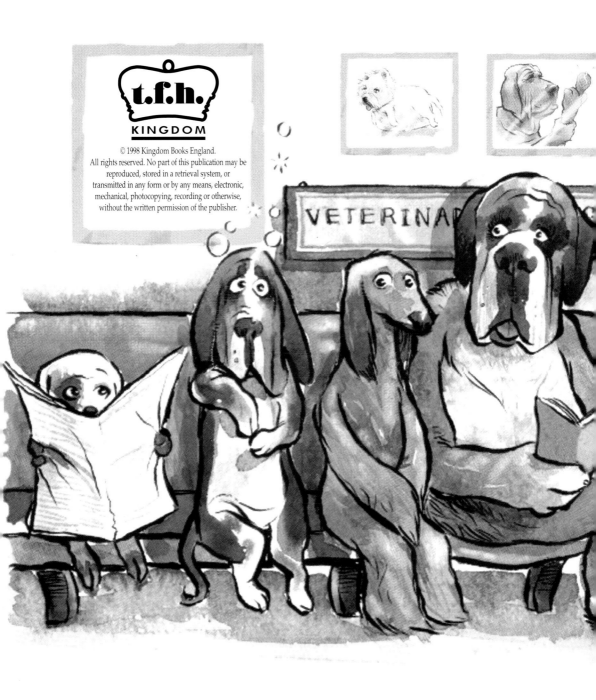

contents

 *preface*

Nearly every time I have suggested homeopathy to treat a dog, I have provoked one of two reactions. Either the clients knew very little about homeopathy or they did not know it could be used to treat animals. This book provides a simple explanation of homeopathy and how it works, with particular reference to dogs. I do not suggest that the book can take the place of the knowledge and skill of the experienced veterinary surgeon, but I have found that homeopathy has a great deal to offer toward the treatment of dogs. I have used it very successfully on clients' dogs and our own family pets. Sometimes I have used homeopathy alone and sometimes I have used it alongside conventional treatments.

The first two chapters of the book describe the history and the basic principles of homeopathy. These principles are vitally important and must be applied when you select remedies for your dog.

The later chapters discuss the treatment of many problems. True homeopathic treatment relies on recognition of the symptoms of the whole patient, and does not seek to make a specific diagnosis of each disease. The descriptions of these symptoms do not make attractive reading, but please don't let that put you off. Hopefully, your dog won't have any of these problems. Certainly, he won't have them all!

Although homeopathic treatment relies on symptoms, I have written about specific diseases. This is to make it easier to recognise the problems, and to talk about them with your vet. In this way, I hope you will be able to use the best of homeopathic medicine as well as the best of conventional medicine to produce the best treatment for your dog.

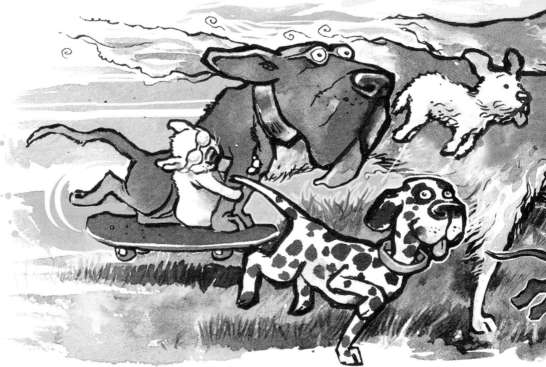

dedication

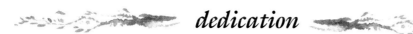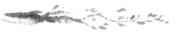

To Christina, my wife, for her untiring love and help in checking and correcting manuscripts, and for sending me back to the word processor when I did not make myself clear!
To Christina ('Charlie'), our daughter, who suggested I write this book.
To Florence, my mother, who, by her example, gave me my understanding of dogs.
Without their help I could not have attempted to write this book.

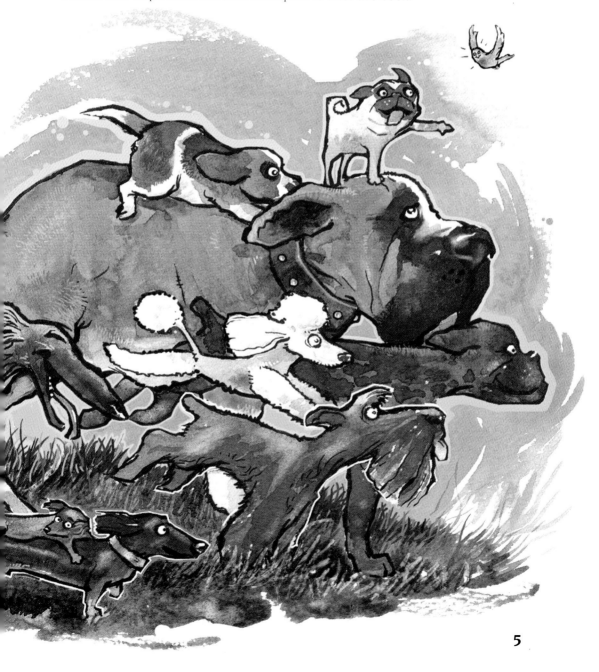

 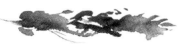

an introduction to homeopathy

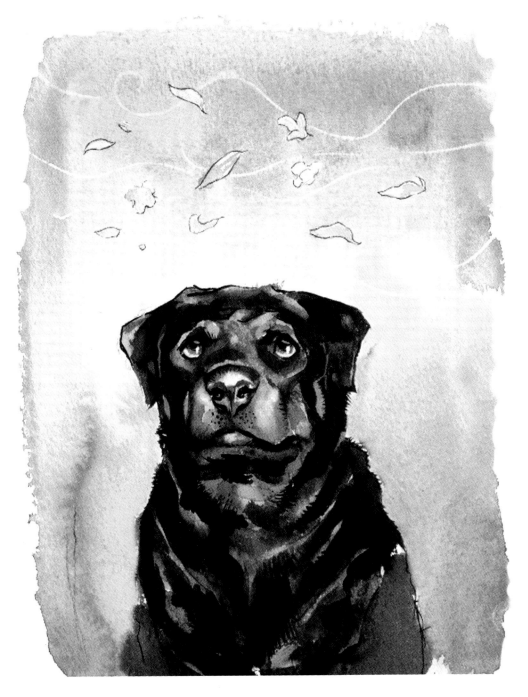

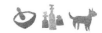

what is homeopathy?

Homeopathy is a system of medical treatment where the patient is treated with substances which, if given in large doses, would produce the symptoms from which the patient is already suffering. Homeopathic remedies are diluted to such an extent that the original substance is non-detectable in the medicine.

What a complicated and mind-blowing statement! How did all this come about?

The principles of homeopathy have cropped up intermittently in medicine since classical Greek times. However, the modern system of homeopathy was established in the late eighteenth century by an Austrian doctor, Samuel Hahnemann. At that time, although the cause of malaria was not known, quinine was being used as a successful treatment. Hahnemann discovered that, by taking very large doses of quinine, he produced symptoms in himself very similar to those of malaria. This led him to think that symptoms caused by a substance in poisonous doses could be cured by the same substance in small doses. He said that like could be cured with like.

He then discovered that very small doses indeed could produce a cure. I suppose there may be a curious logic to this. If large doses of quinine produced the symptoms of malaria, and smaller doses cured malaria, even smaller doses of quinine may make an even stronger remedy. In terms of the power to cure, 'less is more'.

Hahnemann went on to produce remedies which contained the substances in infinitely small doses. He experimented on himself, his family and friends, giving poisonous substances and observing the symptoms that these produced. He noted the symptoms produced in all parts of the body, and also any changes in behaviour. This he called 'proving' the remedy. He must have had a very trusting circle of friends to allow him to dose them with potential poisons!

He also noted any effects on the symptoms produced by external factors, such as: changes in the weather, hot or cold surroundings, different times of the day, or whether the symptoms were worse for resting or moving. He noted whether the symptoms were better or worse for these changes. In all he produced over 60 remedies by experimenting and recording in detail the symptoms that these substances produced. Since that time many more remedies have been proven.

To prepare the remedy, the original substance is diluted in successive stages. This is usually done by diluting one part of the substance in one hundred parts of diluent. Then the diluted substance is diluted again one part in one hundred parts of diluent. Between each stage the remedy is shaken vigorously. A commonly-used remedy might have gone through six of these stages. Its strength, or Homeopathic Potency, would be shown as 6c. In some countries this is shown as 6cH (centesimal Hahnemannienne).

If the dilutions had been one in ten the potency is shown as 6x, or D6. Mathematically the potency 6c means that the dilution of the substance is 1/1000000000000! As the number of dilutions increases the remedy becomes stronger. Therefore a remedy which has a potency of 30c is stronger than one of 6c.

The theoretical problem with all this is the tremendous dilution of the original substances. The mathematicians tell us there is not a single molecule of the original substance left in the remedy. I am not a mathematician but, if I put a pea in a bucket of water, and then take out a teaspoonful of the water, it is most unlikely that I will remove the pea. That is the kind of dilution we are talking about!

So, if there is nothing in the remedy, how does homeopathy work? It seems that the vigorous shaking of each dilution is essential for the production of the remedy. Does this create some sort of electrical charge, or electromagnetic pattern, which is transferred from the substance into the liquid?

Ancient Chinese philosophers suggested that the things that are useful in life are not always as they appear. For example, if we make a glass bottle, it is not the bottle which is useful. The useful thing is the space in the bottle. We can put something in the space. Without that space, the glass of the bottle would be useless. Often, the essential things of life are invisible to our eyes. The useful part of a homeopathic remedy is something we cannot see or touch.

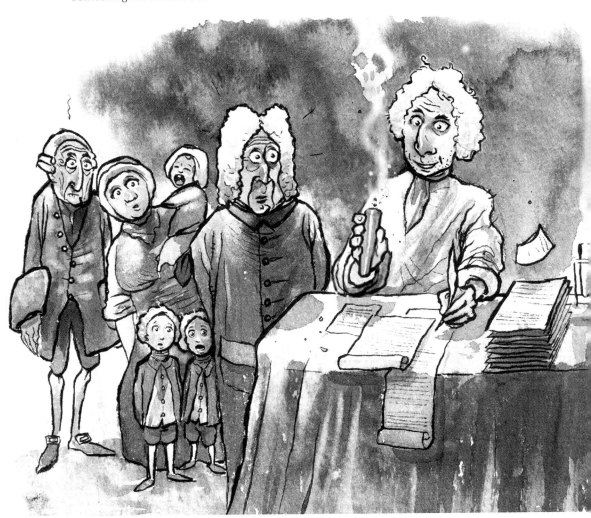

Samuel Hahnemann observed the effects of poisons on his own body – as well as family and friends!

We know that cortisone prevents homeopathic remedies working. One of the actions of cortisone is to prevent the immune system from working. Is this why it stops homeopathy being effective?

The immune system is very complicated. Put very simply, it recognises an intrusion by a foreign organism, such as a bacterium or a virus, and produces specific 'white' blood cells which link up with the invading organism. Then the whole lot is destroyed, absorbed by other large white cells. The immune system appears to remember the invasion by a particular infectious agent, such as the distemper virus, and can respond very quickly if the infection appears again. This is how immunity to a disease is acquired naturally. The mechanisms for this process are, of course, very complicated. Is there some other mechanism which we do not understand that enables the immune system to respond to homeopathic remedies?

Again, we do not really understand how the body heals itself. If we cut a finger, the wound heals and the finger is the same as ever. Why does the skin grow across in the same way as before?

If we break a bone, the tissues around the fracture lay down bony tissues to make the fracture immobile. (We help this process by applying a splint or plaster cast.) The bone then heals. Cells produce bone which re-establishes the original structure of the bone. Why does this happen?

The most likely explanation is that the healing process is controlled by the genetic make-up of the cells. Different parts of the body have different genes 'switched on'. Do they control the renewal of specific tissues in original shapes? After all, the creation of the body was originally governed by the genes in the cells. Does homeopathy work by stimulating the genes to restore the body to its original healthy state?

We have to be humble. We do not know how homeopathy works. We have to accept that we do not know everything about this world we live in.

All too frequently, conventional medicines are used to suppress symptoms rather than cure them. For example, we use pain killers to suppress pain, and purgatives for constipation. For diarrhoea we use medicines which slow the bowel movements, or bind the gut contents. They do not cure the complaint; they mask the symptoms. It seems that homeopathic remedies stimulate the body to return to its natural healthy state. The symptoms are not suppressed, they are cured.

Homeopathy is so safe because the remedies are diluted to infinitesimal amounts. The remedies do not produce side effects as do conventional medicines. They can be used intermittently, for long periods of time, to treat chronic or recurring diseases.

However, because we cannot explain scientifically how homeopathy works, and in theory the remedy does not contain any substance, many people are sceptical. Some people have tried to explain the success of homeopathy by suggesting that it is all in the mind of the patient. People believe they will be cured, so their minds condition their bodies to respond. Obviously this cannot be true of animals. They do not know what they are being given, but they respond very well to homeopathic treatments.

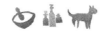
how to use homeopathy

Homeopathy can be used to cure a very large number of problems which can affect your dog. However, I am not suggesting that you dispense with the services of your vet and treat every possible problem with homeopathic remedies. Your vet has had many years of training in understanding the problems of healthy and sick dogs. This training, and his experience in diagnosing, understanding and treating sick dogs is invaluable. Also, although homeopathy treats the symptoms, you should know what your dog's problem is. Then you know how serious the problem is and what kind of help you may need. It is impossible for a single book to replace the knowledge and experience of your vet. Later in this chapter I discuss how you can approach your vet about using homeopathy (see page 18).

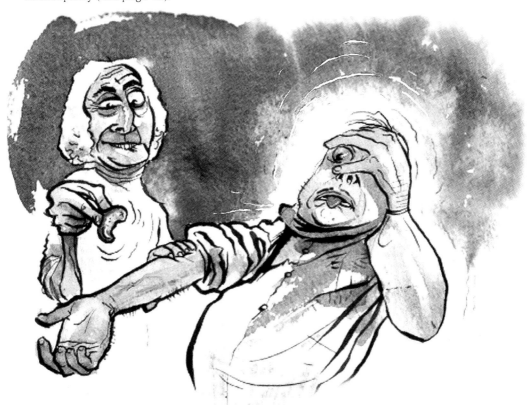

Bleeding the patient was a traditional method in the 1800s.

Originally, those practising homeopathic medicine in humans thought that it was not possible to combine homeopathy with treatment by conventional methods. This was probably partly due to the infighting and war of words and insults going on between homeopaths and conventional doctors. Also, at that time, some 200 years ago, archaic methods were being used, such as bleeding the patient. We know now that such treatment was definitely detrimental to the sufferer!

Homeopathy can be used alongside many modern drugs. In treating our dogs we can have the best of both worlds. If your dog has an acute infection, it makes sense to use antibiotics to suppress the infection. The body then, hopefully, repairs the ravages to the body tissues caused by the infection. If we add treatment with homeopathic remedies based on the symptoms shown, we can stimulate the body to return to its normal, healthy state more quickly and more completely. It is in this kind of way that the two methods of treatment can be combined to help each other.

Having said that, I do admit that life is not entirely that simple. First, there are drugs which appear to interfere with the action of homeopathic remedies. The most important are the group of drugs called corticosteroids (cortisone). One of the actions of these drugs is to depress the immune system. It is possible that homeopathy works through some unknown mechanism of the immune system (see chapter 1). Homeopathy may not work because the immune system has been depressed by the corticosteroids.

It appears that the group of drugs called anti-histamines may also interfere with homeopathy because of their action on the immune system.

Sometimes modern drugs produce undesirable side effects. You can treat these with a remedy made from the offending drug. The drug is diluted in exactly the same way as in the preparation of other homeopathic remedies. You are treating the symptoms caused by the drug with the same drug in homeopathic potency. Once again, you are treating like with like.

If homeopathy is new to you, I suggest that you begin by treating the local problems which are not serious or life threatening. Leave the diagnosis and treatment of the big, serious problems to the experience and knowledge of your vet. You can support his treatment with homeopathic remedies. Also, you may be able to sort out any problems which remain after conventional treatment has finished. After all, you do want the best treatment and the minimum of suffering for your dog. As your knowledge and experience of homeopathy increase, I am sure you will find yourself using it more and more for any problems your dog may have.

The Remedies
The remedies are known by their old-fashioned Latin names. In this book I have used the full Latin names but in practice often abbreviations are used which make it easier to label bottles and talk about the remedies. For example, the name for the remedy made from bee venom is *Apis Mellifica*, and this is often called *Apis Mel*. The remedy made from Poison Ivy, *Rhus Toxicodendron*, is commonly referred to as *Rhus Tox*.

Please do not be put off by these apparently formidable Latin names. They may seem very difficult at first, but you will be surprised how quickly they become familiar friends. In the Section II, where individual problems are discussed, the Latin names are in **bold** type. This will help you recognise the names more quickly.

Choosing a Remedy
First of all you need to understand the principles of treating with homeopathy. Homeopathy is a system which is intended to treat the whole patient (in this case, your dog). To choose a remedy you must take into account the symptoms your dog shows,

his personality and his physical characteristics. For example, he may be excitable, aggressive, or gentle and affectionate. He may be fat and lazy, or thin and hyperactive. His normal mental state may have been altered by some recent event, or by his problem. With humans, it is possible to ask the patient about his symptoms and gain a very accurate picture of them – providing the patient tells the truth, that is. Obviously, you cannot ask your dog, but at least he cannot lie to you. You have to use your own powers of observation about his problem, then, after thinking about the immediate problem, you have to look beyond it. You have to become a detective. This is interesting, a challenge and fun. When you cure your dog, it is very rewarding.

It is easy to assess some things, such as the character and colour of a discharge, such as a nasal discharge or diarrhoea. It is more difficult to relate the symptoms to outside factors, such as whether they are worse for movement, or at night. It is even more difficult to understand your dog's reaction to his problem, or whether the problem has been caused by some apparently unrelated event.

Perhaps an example of a real case will help to illustrate what I am saying. Bosun is a three-year-old Golden Retriever who was brought to the surgery with eczema. He had numerous sores. Examination of his skin and all the tests did not suggest a reason for the problem. Anti-inflammatory drugs relieved the itchiness so that he stopped biting himself. However, as soon as the drugs were stopped, the problem started all over again. The drugs were simply suppressing the symptoms and were not curing the problem.

Then one day I saw him in his home, not at the surgery. Bosun greeted me like a long-lost friend, as Retrievers do, and brought me a toy. A minute or two later he went out into the small garden. While talking to his owner, I noticed Bosun sitting on the grass, staring at a blank wall. He did not seem to be noticing anything, nor listening, nor smelling. He just sat! I asked his owner if this was his usual behaviour. She told me he had sat like that ever since they had moved to the house a few months before. She then told me that she thought Bosun missed her husband who had died the year before.

Then I suggested homeopathic treatment. The owner was willing to try anything. I prescribed Ignatia 30c for three to five days. After three days the dog had stopped biting himself. Within 10 days all the skin sores had healed. The problem did not recur. Bosun's skin problem had been caused by his grief over losing his owner and moving house. Not only had the Ignatia cured the grief, it also cured the symptoms of the skin problem. In addition, I think that Ignatia suits the nature of the Golden Retriever, which is a sensitive dog with changeable moods, ranging from furious excitement to profound introspection.

So how do you decide what remedy to give your dog? Homeopathy is a system which tries to treat the whole animal, not just one bit of him. You look at the symptoms of your dog's problem, and choose one or more remedies for those symptoms. You also try to look at your dog objectively, and decide what his personal qualities are. It may help to ask other people who know your dog well. Ask them about the character of your dog. Is he affectionate or aggressive? Is he obedient? Is he is too fat or too thin? Is he lazy or greedy? After they have given their opinions about your dog, I hope your friends will still be your friends!

Please don't think that I am suggesting your dog is full of vices. It is just that it is most important that you assess what he is like, both as a character and physically.

Another principle to remember is that, because the remedy you choose is tailored to the individual dog, you may use different remedies to treat a similar problem in different dogs, or on different occasions. Also, you may use a remedy to treat one condition on one occasion, and then use the same remedy to treat an entirely different problem at another time. Now, I have subjected you to yet another complicated statement!

Let us look at another example. Let us imagine that your dog has been given antibiotics for a nasal discharge. He is much better but he still has a discharge of creamy, yellow pus from his nostrils. Probably he has a chronic sinusitis (an infection of the sinuses, or cavities, in the face bones). These sinuses drain into the nose. If you refer to the section on Nose Problems (page 66), you will find the remedies I suggest for treating nasal discharges. From this list you may decide Pulsatilla 30c is the appropriate remedy. You may feel this is confirmed by your dog being gentle and affectionate.

If you look up Pulsatilla in the section on the Remedies, you will see that it helps problems which are worse indoors in a warm room. All this fits together very nicely, so you give your dog Pulsatilla 30c, one tablet twice a day. After three days the discharge has disappeared completely. That may well be the end of the problem.

Alternatively, your dog may start to have a nasty green discharge from his nose. What has gone wrong? The answer, probably, is nothing. Then you remember that the discharge was green before the treatment with antibiotics. The antibiotics suppressed the original infection but did not cure it, and your dog developed the chronic creamy, yellow discharge which you have cured. The problem has reverted to its original form, the green discharge.

Now you may decide to treat with Mercurius Solubilis 6c, a remedy which is indicated for a green nasal discharge which may be worse in a warm room. This may produce a cure, and the problem disappears completely.

Obviously it is easy for me to produce a neat, hypothetical case like this. However, it does illustrate the kind of thinking, and the changes in treatment you may have to adopt, in order to use homeopathy successfully.

To summarise how you approach choosing a remedy: you have to think beyond the immediate problem which is worrying you, and assess your dog as a whole. You should take note of:

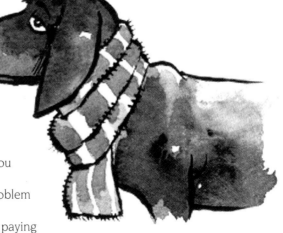

1 the characteristics of the problem which you think requires treatment
2 the characteristics of any other minor problem which your dog may have
3 the character and behaviour of your dog, paying particular attention to any changes from his normal behaviour

A nasal discharge is easy to diagnose.

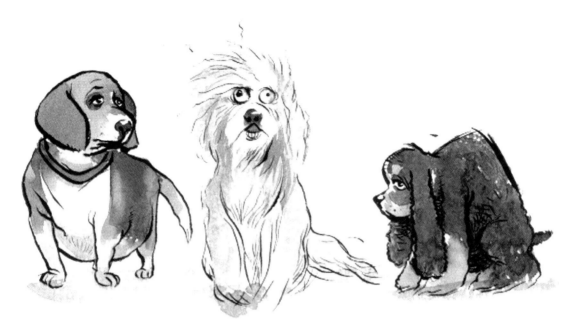

To use homeopathy successfully, it is important to know what your dog is like.

4 situations that make the symptoms worse, for example, the symptoms may be worse when it is hot, or for movement, or at night
5 any previous treatment for the problem
6 how long the problem has been going on, and whether it relates to any earlier illness or incident in the dog's life.

Choosing the Potency
The potency of homeopathic remedies is described in chapter 1. You will remember that it is a measure of the dilution of the remedy and, hence, its strength. The greater the number of serial dilutions, the stronger, or more potent, the remedy. The potency of a remedy which has been made by making a dilution of 1/100 is 1c, or 1cH. If this remedy is subjected to a series of further dilutions, each one being 1/100, a more dilute and stronger remedy is produced. If the remedy is diluted in this way six times, it is called 6c or 6cH. Thirty dilutions produces a remedy of 30c or 30cH, and a thousand dilutions is 1M. A dilution of 6c is 1/1000,000,000,000, and a dilution of 1M is a dilution of 1/1 with 2000 noughts added!

The hundredfold, or centesimal, dilutions are the ones most commonly used. Sometimes remedies of very low potency are made by making the dilutions in tenfold stages. Three such dilutions would be written as 3x or D3. The only remedy of such a strength suggested in this book is Urtica Urens 3x. It reduces the production of milk in the bitch, and examples of its use can be found in the sections on pregnancy and the female dog.

It seems that the higher potencies have a narrower, but more powerful, field of action than the lower potencies. If your assessment of the suitable remedy is very accurate, it may be better to choose a high potency. If you are less sure of your choice

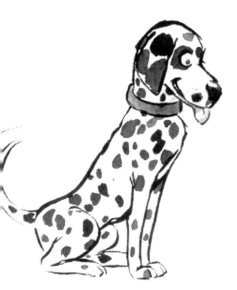

of remedy, use a lower potency. Using a high potency is like using a fierce small jet from a hose. It has a big effect over a very small area. Lower potencies are more like using a spray. They have a less powerful action, but cover a wider area.

In this book I have suggested potencies which you can use for treating the various symptoms. However, unlike the strength of conventional tablets, the potency required is not necessarily the same for each case. In general, I suggest that higher potencies, in more frequent doses, are better for acute symptoms. Lower potencies, in more infrequent doses, are more useful for chronic, longstanding problems. However, if a chronic problem is not responding, and you are sure you have the right remedy, you may find that changing to a higher potency, with infrequent dosing, produces the cure.

Dosing: How Often and for How Long?

Like potencies, dosing may vary from case to case. In general I advise you to dose twice daily for three to five days. Stop the treatment when the symptoms disappear. This may mean you only have to give one or two doses. In very acute cases, and where there is a great deal of pain, hourly dosing may be needed. In chronic, longstanding cases, I suggest more infrequent dosing, such as once or twice a week. With this infrequent dosing, you may have to write down when the next dose is due. In all cases, you should stop giving the remedy as soon as the symptoms disappear.

With chronic cases it is most important not to dose too often. A chronic problem may have been there a long time, and it is only reasonable to expect that it will take time for your dog's body to become healthy again. In chronic cases, dose at infrequent intervals, and give the remedy time to work. This is another reason why I suggest that, if you are new to homeopathy, you should begin by treating the simpler problems first. In that way you can gain experience and confidence.

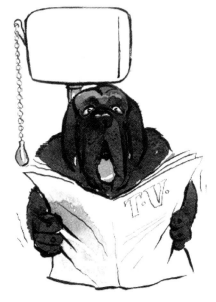

Get to know your dog's daily routine.

Buying Remedies

Veterinary surgeons practising homeopathy will have a large selection of suitable remedies. Normally, when treating your dog, the vet will be able to provide the recommended remedy.

How do you buy the remedies yourself? Nowadays, in the United Kingdom, many pharmacies and health food shops stock a limited number of homeopathic remedies. These are likely to be those which are frequently used. Nearly always they are in the 6c potency. If the remedy you need is not in stock, it is very likely that the shop can obtain it for you from their supplier.

I have already explained there are an enormous number of remedies available. In this book, I have tried to confine my recommendations to a limited number of remedies. Even so, I have suggested using more than 70. Although the individual remedies are relatively inexpensive, it would be very expensive and a waste of money to buy them all. Most of them you would never use. Below are some suggested remedies which you might like to buy as a 'starter' and emergency kit. If your dog already has a problem you may wish to add the appropriate remedy to this list.

Arnica Montana 30c and **Aconitum Napellus 30c** are the basic remedies for treating bruising and shock from injuries. Do try to get these in the 30c potency. In emergencies, I find that this works even more dramatically than the 6c potency.

Also consider buying:
Bryonia Alba
Apis Mellifica
Hypericum Perforatum
Rhus Toxicodendron

Usually these four remedies are readily available in the 6c potency.

Storing and Using the Remedies

It is generally advised that homeopathic remedies are handled and used with special precautions. These precautions are recommended in order to protect the remedies, not you! Many of them may not be necessary. But, until we understand better the nature of the remedy, and how it works, it must be wiser to use the methods and take the precautions which have been successful over the years.

The remedies should be stored carefully in their original containers. They should be kept away from strong light and not be exposed to high temperatures. Please do not leave them out in the full heat of the midsummer sun. They should not be stored close to a substance with a strong smell, such as camphor, mothballs, Vick or oil of eucalyptus. The remedies may become contaminated and made useless by these substances.

When using the remedies, only open one container at a time. If more than one container is open, the remedies may contaminate each other and be altered.

Also, to avoid contamination, remove the tops of the remedies only when you want to extract a tablet. Do not leave the lids off. Remove the tablets by shaking them into your hand. Please, do not put your fingers in the pot. If extra tablets come out of the pot do not replace them.

16

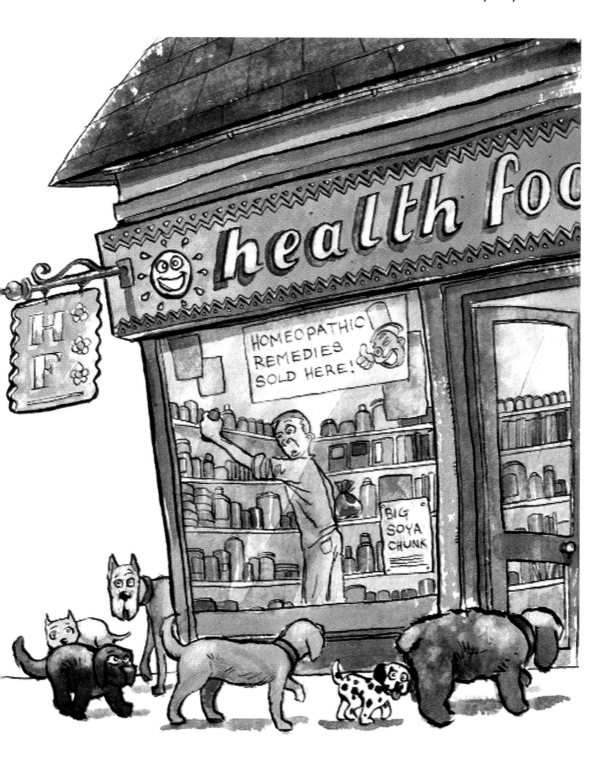

Many health food shops and pharmacies stock homeopathic remedies.

Remedies are available in the form of powders, spherical pillules and small flat tablets. In most cases I have found the tablets easiest to handle when dosing dogs. If you need a powder, you can crush the tablet between two clean teaspoons immediately before dosing your dog. Place the tablet in the bowl of one spoon, then place the back of the second spoon over the tablet. Crush the tablet by squeezing the two spoons together. The crushed remedy can be absorbed through the lining of the mouth, without your dog having to swallow the powder.

It is said that the remedy should be given in a 'clean' mouth, which is not contaminated by food. In human medicine, it is suggested that at least half an hour should elapse between eating and taking the remedy. In fact, the tablets are slightly sweet so many dogs will eat them like a sweet, and it is easy to dose them without food. Having said this, frequently the only way of getting your dog to take the remedy is in food. If you have to do this, I suggest using a bland food such as bread or unsalted butter. In my experience the remedies still work perfectly well.

Vets and Homeopathy

Well, how do you approach your vet over the subject of homeopathy? The first thing is to ask his opinion of homeopathy.

Some will reject it as a load of rubbish. Some will admit they do not know much about the subject, but are happy that you try to use it alongside their conventional treatment. Then you may have to explain, tactfully, that corticosteroids and antihistamines may interfere with homeopathic treatment. With a chronic, longstanding problem, the vet may agree to you trying homeopathy instead of conventional treatment.

Some vets will be using homeopathy to a greater or lesser extent already. These vets will be very interested in helping you find the right remedy for your dog.

If your vet does not use homeopathy, you have to decide whether you want to 'go it alone' in selecting a remedy for your dog, or whether you want to seek the opinion of a vet who uses homeopathy. In either case, you will find the information in this book very useful. If you treat the dog yourself and produce an effective cure, you may help convince your own vet that homeopathy does work.

If you want the help of another vet you should use the system commonly called referral. This means that your vet knows that you are going to take the dog to another practice. He may recommend you to a vet he knows who uses homeopathy. Your vet provides this second vet with a complete history of your dog's problem. He will give his diagnosis, what treatment your dog has had, and the results of any tests which may have been made. The new vet will tell your vet his assessment of the case, and what treatment he has given your dog. In this way, both vets know exactly how your dog is being treated. This must be in the best interests of your dog. The vet advising on homeopathy may not be conveniently near you. If some emergency occurs, your own vet will know what treatment your dog is receiving.

Please do not be embarrassed or worried about asking for a second opinion. It is normal, professional practice to seek the opinion of someone who specialises in a particular subject or treatment. In human medicine you would expect to see a specialist consultant about a skin or hip problem. You are the client and are paying for the treatment. In the same way, your dog is entitled to the best treatment you can afford.

How do you find a vet who practises homeopathy? The best way is by a personal recommendation from someone you know. You may find a vet offering homeopathic treatment in your local Yellow Pages. You can get a list of Homeopathic Vets from the British Association of Homeopathic Veterinary Surgeons (see Useful Addresses).

Incidentally, if your dog is terrified of going to the vet's surgery, try giving him two doses of Silicea 6c, starting about an hour before the appointment.

Treating Your Dog Yourself

I hope that, having read this far, you will now want to try homeopathy for any problems which your dog may have. When using the recommended remedies in this book, please remember, and refer to, the points and explanations which I have already made. To get the best results from homeopathy, remember that you need to treat more than the symptoms of the immediate problem. You must consider any other problems which, although trivial, may be present as well. Also, you must remember to think of your dog's character and his physical condition.

In the next section of this book, I have written about many of the problems which dogs can have and I have divided them into sections on different parts of the body. This should help you to find the particular problem which your dog may have.

Having found the problem, you will find possible remedies listed in alphabetical order, together with the symptoms they can be expected to cure. Many of the symptoms described are unpleasant and, to say the least, colourful! These descriptions are really necessary. Perhaps I should recommend that it is better not read these parts of the book over the breakfast table or at bedtime!

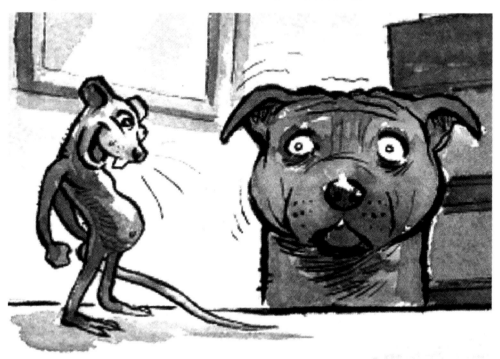

Even a nervous dog can be helped with homeopathic remedies.

Having found one or more remedies which seem suitable for your dog's problem, please refer to the next part of the book which describes all the remedies recommended in the book. The principal actions of each remedy are given, and also listed are the other parts of the body which that particular remedy can help.

I have suggested potencies for each problem and these are the ones I have found the most useful. If you have the remedy in a different potency, it may be better to try that potency rather than delay treatment. This general advice does not apply to Urtica Urens in the control of milk formation. If you want to dry up milk, you must use a very low potency. To encourage milk, use a high potency.

This is where your detective work comes in. Does your dog have any other minor problems? Is the remedy recommended for that part of the body? Look in the section on that part of the body, and see if your chosen remedy is right for these minor symptoms. Think back to when the problem started. Does it relate to an illness or an event in the dog's life? You may find a different remedy, which is suitable for more than one problem.

Also, bear in mind the type of dog for which the remedy is recommended. A remedy which fits the entire make-up of your dog, called a Constitutional Remedy, is the most powerful treatment you have in homeopathy. It treats the whole dog, not just the symptoms of the problems which have arisen.

If you are not able to find a Constitutional Remedy, do not despair! Use the remedy which is most suitable for the symptoms your dog is showing. You will almost certainly get some improvement in these symptoms. You may also get new symptoms because there is a previous, underlying problem. Earlier in this chapter I described a nasal discharge turning from a creamy colour to green. In this hypothetical case, the dog had been treated by conventional medicine. However, it is a good example of a problem which, having been treated homeopathically on symptoms alone, reverted to an earlier problem.

If the symptoms appear to change, be prepared to change the remedy.

I would like to remind you of the six, very basic principles to consider when choosing a remedy. You should take note of:

1 the characteristics of the problem which you think requires treatment
2 the characteristics of any other minor problem which your dog may have
3 the character and behaviour of your dog, paying particular attention to any changes from his normal behaviour
4 situations that make the symptoms worse. For example, the symptoms may be worse when it is hot, when the dog moves, or at night
5 any previous treatment for the problem
6 how long the problem has been going on, and whether it relates to any earlier illness or incident in the dog's life.

 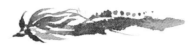

the problems

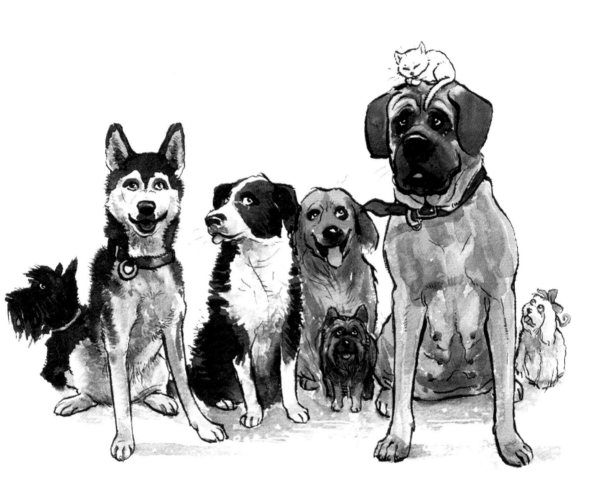

anal area

Anal glands

Anal glands are scent glands, and there is one on each side of the anus. Normally they are emptied when the dog is frightened. Like the foul-smelling secretion given off by foxes and skunks, the smell from a dog's anal glands is meant to deter an enemy. When the glands become too full, they empty automatically as a motion is passed. Sometimes they become blocked, swollen and painful. The dog bites his tail. He may drag his bottom along the ground and on the carpets. Also, the glands may fail to empty in cases of chronic diarrhoea. Manual emptying relieves the pain. The glands are often removed surgically in chronic cases.

The glands may become infected. These infections are difficult to cure completely with antibiotics. Homeopathic treatment can be helpful when there is chronic infection, or the problem occurs frequently. I recommend giving:

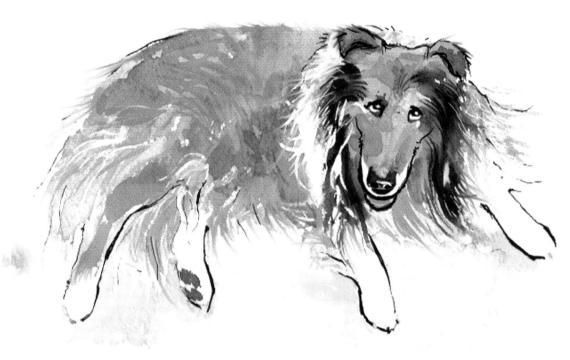

Any infection will make your pet feel unhappy.

Hepar Sulphuris Calcareum 30c when there is white, foul-smelling pus in the glands. The glands may be very painful.

Sanicula 6c is indicated when there is a brown, foul and fishy-smelling discharge from the glands.

Silicea 6c when there is scar tissue around the glands. Over a period of time it helps the elimination of pus from the damaged glands.

Anal tumours

These are tumours in the area around the anus. They start as quite small, hard swellings, but can grow together to become large, infected and smelly malignant masses. Because they occur in the older male dog, they are often treated by dosing the patient with female hormones. They are also treated conventionally by surgical removal or by cryosurgery, which means killing the tissue by freezing it. However the tumours often recur. Homeopathy can be used alone to relieve this problem, but is also very helpful when combined with conventional treatment.

I suggest using:

Calcarea Fluorica 30c to reduce the size of the tumours. It is useful in the early stages when the tumours are small and hard, and if larger tumours are bleeding.

Nitricum Acidum 30c helps when there is ulceration and bleeding close to the anus itself.

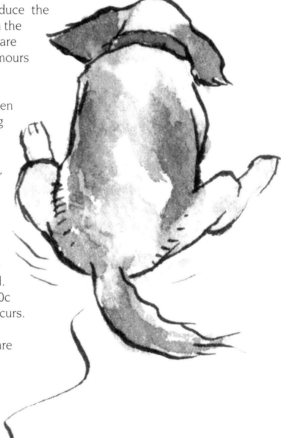

Thuja Occidentalis 6c will, over a period of time, help to reduce and control the tumours. I recommend one tablet twice daily for five days and then one tablet twice a week. Stop treatment when the tumour has been reduced. Repeat treatments with Thuja 30c are needed where the tumour recurs.

Further treatments for tumours are discussed in the section on Tumours and Warts (page 92).

Blocked anal glands may cause your dog to bob-sleigh
across the carpet.

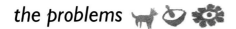

the back

While fractures of the bones of the spine can occur, most back problems in dogs are associated with injury to joints of the spine. Fractures can be detected from X-rays and need specialist surgical attention.

Injured spinal joints are very painful. There may be prolapse of the disc which forms a pad between the vertebrae, commonly called a 'slipped disc'. Swelling around the injury, or the slipped disc, may put pressure on the neighbouring nerves causing paralysis, particularly of the hind legs. Homeopathy is very helpful if given as soon as possible after the injury. Homeopathic remedies may be given while more sophisticated diagnosis and treatment is being organised, and often cure the problem by themselves.

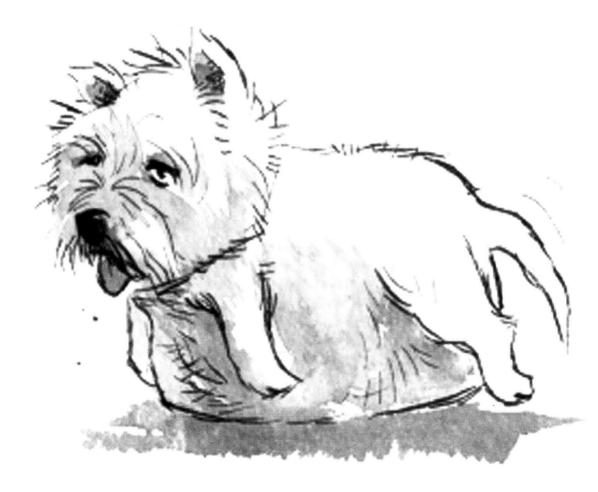

Obesity can cause back problems; as well as a diet, try Calacarea Carbonica 30c.

I suggest:

Arnica Montana 30c as soon as the injury appears. Swelling, pain and pressure on the nerves is reduced by this remedy, and it can cure the problem by itself. I recommend one tablet every 15 minutes for four doses, and then one tablet four times a day.

Other remedies can be given, chosen according to the symptoms:

Aconitum Napellus 30c when the dog is in a state of shock, or is very distressed by the condition.

Apis Mellifica 6c for the dog who has lost control over passing stools.

Berberis Vulgaris 6c when there is pain in the lower back. Urine may be scanty and difficult to pass.

Bryonia Alba 30c when symptoms are worse for exercise and heat.

Calacarea Carbonica 30c if the dog is very fat or indolent.

Causticum 6c when, because of the injury, the dog is not able to pass urine and motions.

Hekla Lava 6c to reduce excessive bone formation at the injury site. Bony lumps can cause pain or paralysis by pressing on nerves.

Hypericum Perforatum 30c when there is a lot of pain. It has a particularly beneficial action on damaged nerves.

Nux Vomica 6c for the dog who passes urine continually and involuntarily, and the dog who is not able to pass motions.

Phosphorus 6c when there is paralysis with pain. It is particularly indicated for the thin dog in poor condition.

Plumbum Metallicum 6c can be used when there is paralysis of the hind quarters. Motions may be hard and black.

Rhus Toxicodendron 30c when symptoms are worse for rest, typically when the dog gets out of bed.

Ruta Graveolens 6c to help repair damage to the ligaments supporting the joints of the back. It will also help to relieve pain in the lower back.

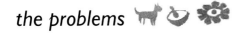

behaviour

Good training is the essential conventional treatment for behaviour problems. Also good training usually prevents bad behaviour in the first place. Homeopathy can be of great help in sorting out problems when they do occur. It can also help to sort out 'hang-ups' that your dog may have, causing fear and excessive excitement. When using these remedies, please remember to adapt your choice to suit your dog's constitution whenever possible.

There are many occasions when giving two remedies can be helpful. For example, if your dog is very jealous of a new pet in the house, and behaves aggressively, you might consider giving both Lachesis and Belladonna.

Aconitum Napellus 30c for a dog who has been badly frightened. It also helps the dog who is afraid of thunder.

Arnica Montana 30c for the dog who is afraid of being approached or touched by people.

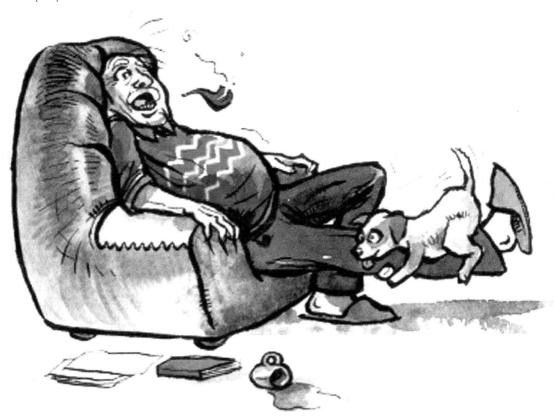

Tarentula Hispana 30c reduces excessive sexual behaviour.

Argentum Nitricum 6c for the dog who is anxious and apprehensive. It is indicated for the elderly dog who seeks reassurance. It is also indicated for the dog who likes company and may become destructive when bored.

Belladonna 30c for the aggressive or excited dog. It is of particular help when the bad behaviour is sudden and violent. If aggression is a result of fear, choose one of the remedies associated with fear.

Borax 6c for the dog who is frightened of sudden noises. It is particularly useful for the gun-shy dog.

Bryonia Alba 30c for the dog who is afraid of movement in any vehicle. It is useful for the dog who roams, and may be used at the same time as a remedy to reduce excessive sexual behaviour.

Calcarea Carbonica 30c for depraved appetite, particularly for the indolent, overweight puppy.

Calcarea Phosphorica 30c also for the dog with a depraved appetite. It works better for the leaner and more active puppy. It is useful for the restless dog, who always wants to be somewhere else.

Chamomilla 30c for the restless and sensitive younger dog or puppy. He may be irritable and may 'lose his temper' easily. It may help with the disobedient dog.

Cinchona Officinalis 6c for the disobedient dog. He may be sulky and indifferent, and resent being touched.

Colocynthis 6c for the irritable dog which is easily offended. It is useful in the dog who is overweight.

Gelsemium Sempervirens 30c for fear and anxiety. It is a useful remedy for the dog who panics, or is frightened by thunder, or by travelling in a car. Also, it can help the dog who is frightened of crowds or being in a Dog Show.

Hyoscyamus Niger 30c is good for the excitable, hysterical dog. He does not like to be left alone, and may be jealous.

Ignatia 30c is a classic remedy for the dog who dislikes being left. This may lead to hysterical destruction of the home. It is also a remedy of choice for the dog suffering from bereavement, for example after a death in the family, or of a companion animal.

Lachesis 30c for the dog who does not like being touched, or who may be very jealous. It may help when a new baby or pet comes into a household.

Lycopodium 30c for the irritable dog who is afraid of being alone.

Nux Vomica 30c for the aggressive dog, who does not like being touched or approached. It is also indicated when digestive disturbances are present.

Phosphoricum Acidum 30c for the young dog. It helps the dog who does not like being left, or is afraid of thunder and other loud noises. It is of particular use for the puppy who panics when separated from his litter mates.

Phosphorus 30c for the dog who is afraid of being left alone, and is frightened of thunder. It can also help with dogs and bitches who are oversexed. It is indicated for dogs with depraved appetite.

Picricum Acidum 6c for the dog who is oversexed.

Pulsatilla 30c for the dog who is shy and afraid of being left, or needs consolation when separated from a companion. It can help dogs who panic. It is particularly indicated in affectionate bitches.

Sepia 30c for the indifferent, irritable dog. It is particularly indicated for bitches.

Silicea 6c for the dog who is frightened of veterinary premises. I recommend giving one dose an hour before the appointment and a second dose just before going to the vet.

Staphyragria 6c for the dog who resents being touched and to being corrected in training.

Tarentula Hispania 30c for the hysterical, oversexed dog.

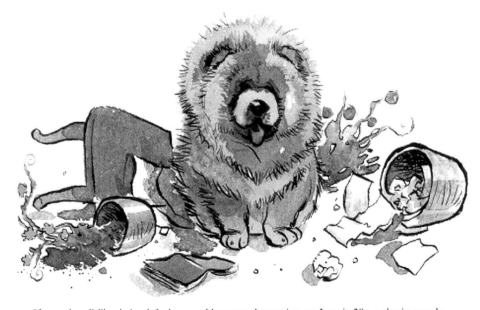

If your dog dislikes being left alone, and becomes destructive, try Ignatia 30c, a classic remedy.

bones

Fractures

Fractures are the most dramatic injuries that happen to bones. The pieces of broken bone must be immobilised so that they can join together and heal. A splint or cast, steel pins or plates, are used. Homeopathy can help the bones to heal more quickly. Immediate homeopathic treatment can help relieve pain and shock from the injury. I recommend using:

Arnica 30c, given as soon as possible. It reduces the swelling and pain around the fracture. I recommend one tablet every 15 minutes for four doses, and then one tablet four times a day until the fracture has been immobilised.

Aconitum Napellus 30c for the dog who is shocked or frightened by the fracture.

After the fracture has been immobilised the following remedies can speed up healing:

Symphytum 30c is the most important remedy to encourage the pieces of bone to knit together.

Calcarea Carbonica 30c to help healing in the fat, indolent dog or puppy.

Calcarea Phosphorica 30c helps bone metabolism. It is useful where a fracture is failing to heal, particularly in the younger, thinner dog.

Calcarea Fluorica 30c helps to harden and strengthen bones. It can be used where the bones are thinner and more porous than normal, a condition called osteoporosis. This problem is more common in older dogs. The thinness of the bones can be seen on the X-ray picture of the fracture.

Various homeopathic remedies can help to heal fractured bones.

Exostoses

Bony lumps, or exostoses, are hard swellings of bone which develop on the surface of bones. Typically they appear around arthritic joints and on bones where the surface has been damaged. Also, sometimes an excessively large lump, called a callus, is left where a broken bone has healed.

To reduce the lump, I suggest:

Hekla Lava 6c is the best remedy to try. I recommend one tablet twice a day for five days, and then one weekly until the swelling reduces.

Calcarea Fluorica 30c can help obstinate cases. Give one tablet twice a day for three days, and then one twice weekly.

Infection or Osteomyelitis
Most infections occur in the soft centre of bones. The bone may become painful and swollen, and eventually pus may burst out it, and through the skin as an abscess. Professional veterinary treatment is needed. X-rays can distinguish between infections and tumours of bones. Also, there are very good antibiotics available for treating bone infections.
Homeopathy can help to speed up the healing process.

Hepar Sulphuris Calcareum 30c as the principal remedy to treat the infection and reduce the pain. It is especially indicated for the very painful bone. Often it speeds up the final removal of infections which are being treated with antibiotics.

Calcarea Carbonica 30c for the younger dog, particularly in the early stages of the problem. It is especially indicated in the fat animal.

Calcarea Phosphorica 30c, also for the younger dog. It is indicated for the thinner animal.

Silicea 30c in the more chronic and less painful cases, when pus is discharging through the skin.

Symphytum 30c to help the healing process. It encourages new bone to develop and replace that destroyed by the infection.

The Younger Dog
Problems for the younger dog are mainly associated with development of the bones.
Rickets occurs in young puppies and usually is the result of faulty feeding. The bones are softer than normal, the legs may bow, and painful swellings may appear near the ends of the bones. These places are, in fact, the places where the bones are growing. Conventional treatment is to give Vitamin D, calcium and other minerals. Homeopathic remedies can help the recovery process enormously.

Calcarea Carbonica 30c to treat the fat, indolent puppy.

Calcarea Phosphorica 30c to encourage healthy bone growth in young dogs. It is particularly indicated for the leaner puppy.

Phosphoricum Acidum 30c to strengthen bones. It is particularly useful in the young dog who has 'outgrown his strength'.

Excessive exercise

Although most puppies seem to have inexhaustible energy, it is very easy to over-exercise the rapidly growing dog. This is particularly true of the larger breeds. Long walks should be avoided. The young dog is so interested in his surroundings that he rushes around too much and for too long. This can cause excessive strain on joints and bones. Please also see the discussion on Hip Dysplasia in the section on Joint Problems (page 55). If your dog is suffering from excessive exercise **Phosphoricum Acidum 30c** can be very helpful.

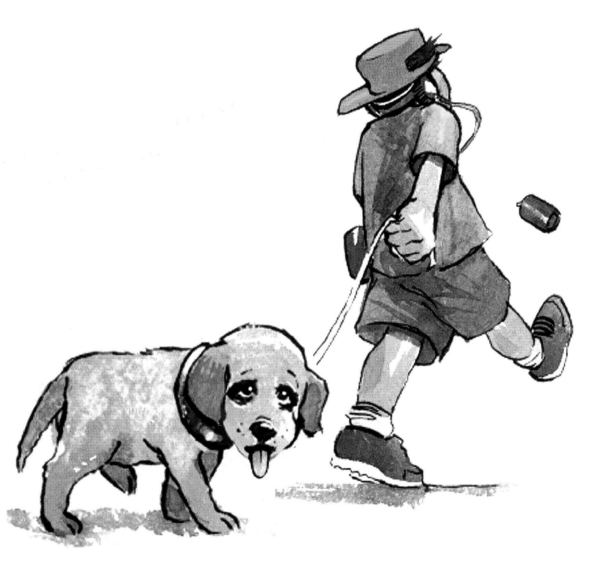

Too much exercise can harm a growing pup's bones and joints.

constipation

There are a number of reasons why a dog may not be able to empty his bowel properly or easily. He may have a temperature. He may have eaten too many bones or he may be dehydrated. He may have damage to his rectum. Older male dogs may have an enlarged prostate gland compressing the rectum (this is discussed in the section on male problems on page 58).

Consequently, constipation varies from being a mild problem to an extremely painful, distressing and serious affliction. If you do not know the reason why your dog is constipated, please ask your vet.

Homeopathy can help relieve the discomfort of constipation, and frequently cures the cause. I recommend using:

Alumina 6c when dog has to strain to pass a stool which may be soft. Often these symptoms are seen in older dogs. In some cases there may be a breakdown in the wall of the rectum, so that faeces become impacted in the hole in the wall. A soft swelling appears in the skin around the anus, and the faeces may have to be removed manually. A surgical repair of the rectal wall may be needed.

Bryonia Alba 6c when stools are large and dark. The dog is uncomfortable and stools are more likely to be passed in the morning.

Carbo Vegetabilis 30c for the dog who passes a lot of offensive wind.

Calcarea Carbonica 6c when the dog has eaten too many bones. The faeces are hard and white. An enema and manual removal of the faeces may also be necessary.

Graphites 6c when the stool is large, hard and comes in a knot held together by mucous threads.

Lycopodium 30c when the stool is hard and small. It is also indicated when there is liver disease.

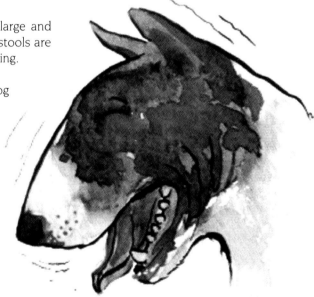

Take the strain!

Nitricum Acidum 30c when the anus is torn or ulcerated.

Nux Vomica 30c when the dog is also vomiting. It is particularly useful when a dog is constipated after an operation.

Sepia 6c when the stools are large and hard. It also useful for the older dog.

Silicea 6c when the stools cannot be completely passed, and may recede back into the rectum. The anus may be very painful.

Sulphur 30c may be given when the stools are large and the anus is red and sore. The dog may have a red, smelly skin.

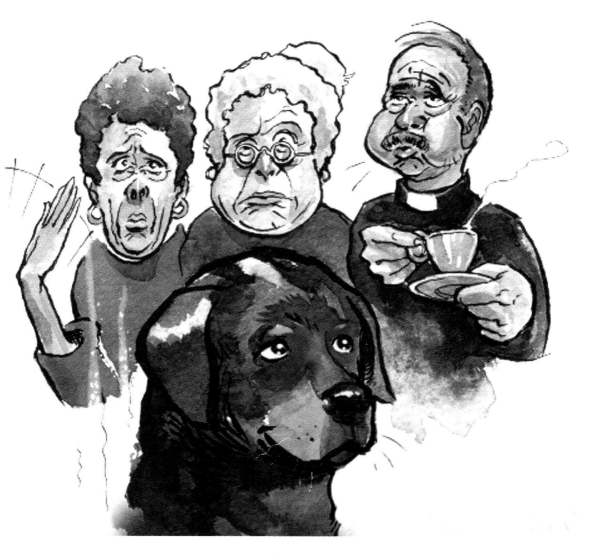

Excessive flatulence can cause social embarrassment for you, if not the dog.

coughing

Coughs are caused by inflammation of the lower respiratory tract, that is the larynx, the windpipe or the lungs. The inflammation may be the result of infection, or of breathing in irritant material, such as dust or a gas.

Coughs can also occur in older dogs suffering from heart disease and congestion of the lungs. These coughs are worse for movement and exercise. Conventionally, infections may be treated with antibiotics, and heart disease with appropriate medicines.

Homeopathy can also be used. The character of the cough and the behaviour of the dog are the most useful guides to the correct remedy. When used at the same time as conventional medicine, homeopathy can reduce the dose of the conventional drug needed to control the cough. In a progressive disease, such as heart problems in an older dog, this leaves room to increase the dose of the conventional drug when it is needed. I recommend:

Aconitum Napellis 6c in the early stages of a coughing problem. It is good for a dry cough after exposure to cold winds. The cough may also be worse at night.

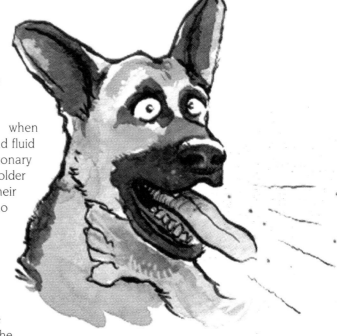

Ammonium Carbonate 6c when breathing is difficult at night, and fluid collects in the lungs (pulmonary oedema). It may also help the older dog whose lungs have lost their elasticity (emphysema), and who has a chronic cough.

Belladonna 30c for a dry cough which is worse at night. The dog may be excited and there may be a change in his bark, due to inflammation of the larynx. Often, it is used with the previous remedy.

Many natural remedies can relieve a harsh cough.

Bryonia Alba 6c when the coughing is worse for movement. The cough is worse in a warm room. The dog may try to take deep breaths between bouts of coughing.

Carbo Vegetabilis 30c for the dog who feels cold and seeks fresh air. His gums may become blue. It is useful for the dog who is very distressed at night.

Causticum 30c for dog who has 'lost his voice'. The bark becomes high-pitched or disappears altogether. Swelling in the larynx has impaired the nerves controlling the voice box. Coughing may be worse in cold winds.

Cinchona Officinalis 6c when the cough is associated with lung disease, such as bronchitis. Breathing may be slow and laboured, and there may be rattling sounds in the chest. The coughing may produce blood.

Drosera 6c when there are frequent spasms of coughing which may produce retching and vomiting.

Hepar Sulphuris Calcareum 30c when there is a painful cough producing pussy mucus. The cough may be worse in cold winds.

Hyoscyamus Niger 30c for a dry spasmodic cough. Often it is worse at night, or when the dog is excited.

Ipecacuanha 30c when there is non-stop coughing. Frequently there is vomiting with the cough. The dog may also cough up blood.

Ledum Palustre 6c when there is coughing and your dog appears short of breath. It helps emphysema, a condition more common in older dogs.

Phosphorus 30c when there is a painful cough. The whole of the dog's body seems to be involved in the effort to cough. It is helpful to the dog with pneumonia who coughs up bloodstained sputum.

Spongia Tosta 6c for a harsh dry cough. The cough may be eased by eating and drinking. It is also a remedy to be given to the dog with heart disease.

Kennel Cough

This is the name given to an infectious cough, which is easily contracted from contact with infected and carrier dogs Kennels provide an ideal environment in which the infection can spread. There are very good vaccines against this disease, and most kennels insist that dogs are vaccinated before taking them in. Please see the section on puppy problems (page 76).

Kennel Cough is a dry, hacking and continuous cough which is very distressing for both dog and owner. It can be cured with antibiotic treatment. Sometimes it takes several days for the cough to go. Treatment with Drosera 6c or Ipecacuanha 6c can be very effective in controlling the cough. Also, please consider giving the other cough remedies in the list above.

diarrhoea

Diarrhoea is usually less life threatening than vomiting, but your dog has a serious problem when the two occur together. Please read the description of dehydration in the section on tummy problems (page 88).

Inflammation of the intestines, the reason why your dog has diarrhoea, may be caused by incorrect feeding or infection. The infection may be local to the intestines themselves, or may be part of a more generalised disease. It is important to find the cause and remove it. Often, changing from a rich food to one less rich, or even from a tinned to a dry food, will resolve the problem. This is particularly true of the larger breeds of dog.

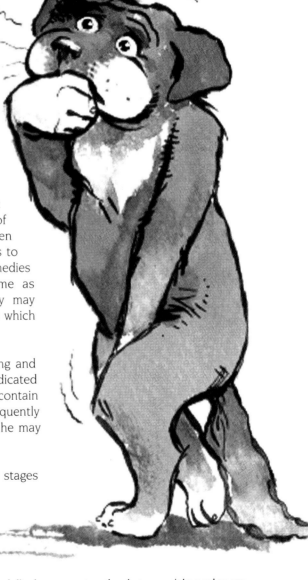

There are many homeopathic remedies for diarrhoea. The nature of the stools, and the behaviour when passing them, are the main symptoms to look for when choosing a remedy. Remedies can also be used at the same time as conventional treatment. Homeopathy may prove particularly useful in conditions which recur frequently.

Arsenicum Album 30c when vomiting and diarrhoea occur together. It is also indicated for smelly, watery stools that may contain blood. The dog is often restless and frequently seeks small quantities of water. Also, he may have a dry, staring coat.

Aconitum Napellum 6c for the early stages of diarrhoea when there is a more generalised infection. It is also useful when the dog has been frightened, or suffered a severe shock.

Try Arsenicum Album 30c when vomiting and diarrhoea occur together, but you might need to use conventional treatment also.

Bryonia Alba 6c when the dog has eaten too much rich food.

Borax 6c for an offensive diarrhoea containing mucous. It is especially indicated in young dogs, or when there is an infection of the mouth and lips.

Carbo Vegetabilis 30c often revives the collapsed dog, even when there appears to be no hope. There may be severe dehydration and the dog may pass a lot of wind.

Chamomilla 30c for a green watery stool which may also contain both yellow and white slime. It is very helpful to the young teething puppy.

Cina Maritima 6c when the stool contains white mucus. The anus may be sore. This remedy is helpful when the problem is associated with worms.

Cinchona Officinalis 6c is a remedy that can be given with other remedies to help restore the dog's strength. It also helps when there is a frothy, yellow and painless stool.

Colocynthis 6c when there is severe pain with the diarrhoea. The dog often shows this by arching his back, and may grunt, grind his teeth, or cry out with the pain.

Gelsemium Sempervirens 30c when diarrhoea is associated with fear or excitement.

Hyoscyamus Niger 30c for involuntary diarrhoea when it is associated with excitement.

Mercurius Corrosivus 30c when the diarrhoea is a forceful, frequent and painful condition. The stool is slimy and may spurt out. There is severe straining.

Mercurius Solubilis 30c for a pasty diarrhoea without much discomfort.

Pulsatilla Nigricans 6c may be used for the shy, affectionate dog and where the stools are variable.

Rhus Toxicodendron 6c when diarrhoea occurs after the dog has been cold and wet. Stools may be slimy, bloody, yellow or frothy. They may be painless, or the dog may strain a lot.

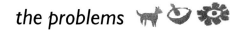

ears

The Ear Canal

Your dog's ear canals can become inflamed, painful and hot for a number of different reasons. There may be excess impacted wax, which may result from an infestation of ear mites or of excess hair growth within the canal. There may be infection producing an offensive discharge. The ear may be constructed so that ventilation of the canal is poor, as is common in Cocker Spaniels. This can lead to an accumulation of wax and to infection. In late summer and autumn dogs frequently get grass seeds in their ears, producing a very sudden and severe pain, with a great deal of head shaking. If you are not absolutely sure of the cause of your dog's problem seek advice from your vet.

Homeopathy can help with all the symptoms, but you must also use conventional methods to remove the cause. Wax needs to be dissolved and antibiotics can be used for infections. Avoid the use of corticosteroids which hinder homeopathic treatment. Mites must be killed with suitable drops. Remember that it is relatively easy to kill the adult mites, but not their eggs. Follow-up treatment, such as a few drops twice weekly, should continue for a month to ensure that all the mites are killed as the eggs hatch.

Hair and grass seeds should be removed. Removal of grass seeds is a job for your vet. Your dog must be anaesthetised because the seeds are so painful. This should be done as soon as possible to relieve the pain and before the seed does too much damage.

Homeopathic remedies can be given according to the symptoms. If the symptoms, such as the nature of the discharge, change, you can switch the treatment to a new remedy. You can also treat with more than one remedy if this seems appropriate. The remedies may not work so well if drops containing steroids have been prescribed.

I suggest you use:

Aconitum Napellus 30c for the early stages, and for the dog who is distressed by the pain. Give one tablet twice a day for one to three days.

Arsenicum Alba 6c when there is a watery discharge. Give one tablet twice a day for five days. Discontinue the treatment if the symptoms disappear earlier.

Belladonna 30c when the ear is hot and swollen. Give one tablet twice daily for a maximum of three days. Often this removes the painful inflammation without the need to give steroids. It helps the dog who is excited and shakes his head, or scratches the ear a lot.

Causticum 30c helps to prevent the development of wax and also helps to remove the wax.

Graphites 6c when there is a chronic, thin and burning discharge. The skin around the ears may be sticky.

Hepar Sulphuris 30c when the ear is very painful to the touch. Give one tablet twice a day until symptoms are gone. This remedy will also be helpful where there is a dark discharge of liquid wax.

Hydrastis Canadensis 30c when there is a thick yellow discharge.

Mercurius Corrosivus 30c when there is a green discharge. Give one tablet twice a day until symptoms disappear. Treat for a maximum of five days.

Pulsatilla 30c when there is a creamy, bland discharge. Give one tablet twice a day for three to five days. This remedy is very useful for the timid and affectionate dog.

Tellurium 30c when there is thickening of the lining to the ear canal. Usually, this is caused by a problem which has been present for a long time. Give one tablet twice a day for three days, then one weekly until the thickening is gone.

Psorinum 200c if your dog has dirty, smelly skin around the ear. Give one tablet twice a day for three doses. There may be delay of seven to ten days before you see any benefit from this treatment so do not use the remedy too frequently. If necessary, the course may be repeated after fourteen days.

The Ear Flap
Ear flaps can become dry and scaly, or swollen, and may be very hot and painful. Whenever there is a problem do look at the ear canal to see that it is healthy. If there is a problem with the canal, this must be treated.

The ear flap can be infested with lice or ticks. Lice are very difficult to see. Usually sucking lice are the ones that are found on the ear flap. They appear as tiny, white translucent creatures, about the size of a pinhead or slightly larger. They attach themselves to the skin, and suck body fluids through the skin. You may see their white eggs, which are often called nits, attached to hairs. Adult lice are easily killed with insecticidal shampoos and lotions. You need to kill the eggs as they hatch. To do this, treat the ear flap every 7–10 days for three weeks.

Ticks suck blood from the dog, and grow into much larger, round creatures. They are best removed individually. Dab them with surgical or methylated spirit and then, after a few seconds, pull them out with a firm tug. This ensures that you remove the head. Please make sure that you are pulling at a tick and not a wart. Your dog won't appreciate you trying to pull off his warts!

Homeopathic treatment can be very helpful in curing the symptoms of ear flap problems. I suggest you use:

Graphites 6c when the ear flap and the surrounding skin is moist and sticky.

Rhus Toxicodendron 6c when the ear flap is inflamed, with intense itching, and there are small vesicles, or blisters, on the inside surface. Give one tablet twice daily until symptoms disappear.

Sulphur 30c in the early stages of a problem. The ear flap is inflamed and red, and the itching is worse in a warm room. Give one tablet twice daily, for up to three days.

Tellurium 30c when the ear flap is thickened, and there is a dry scaly skin. Give one tablet twice daily for three days and then once weekly until the problem is cured. There may also be thickening of the ear canal.

39

Aural Haematoma

The inside of your dog's ear flap may suddenly become swollen, and he may shake his head a lot. The swelling is in fact blood from a blood vessel broken by excessive head shaking. This is called an aural haematoma. Treatment must, of course, include removing the cause of the head shaking, whether the problem is in the ear canal or on the ear flap.

Conventional treatment is to leave the ear flap alone for a few days, while the blood vessel seals itself, and stops bleeding. The swelling is then drained surgically, with the dog anaesthetised. Then the wound is stitched so that it is slightly open, and continues to drain. It takes ten to fourteen days to heal.

Homeopathic treatment can be very successful without the need for this painful and distressing surgery. I recommend:

Arnica Montana 30c Give one tablet every 15 minutes for four doses, then one twice a day for three days. This stops the bleeding. The pressure within the swelling decreases rapidly, and the pain is relieved. Then give

Hamamelis Virginica 6c Dose with one tablet twice daily for three days, followed by a course of one tablet once daily for about a month. This will remove the remaining blood fluids and the blood clot.

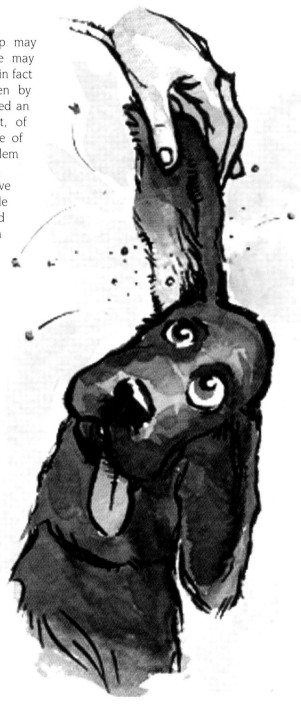

Ear mites can cause painful inflammation. Make sure that both adults and eggs are killed.

eyes

Your dog suddenly has a painful eye. It may be closed and swollen. Tears may be running down his face. He may have one or all of these symptoms. What is the problem? Has he got something in his eye, or ingrowing eyelashes? Are his tear ducts blocked or is his eye damaged? Is he in the early stages of some disease, such as distemper?

Maybe he has a cloudy eye. Is this caused by damage to the surface of the eye? Is there infection within the eye itself? Is it a cataract?

Although many eye problems respond extremely well to homeopathic treatment, diagnosis and understanding the problem are very difficult. Failure to provide the correct treatment can end in disaster. Therefore, I recommend an examination by your vet whenever eye problems occur. But do not despair. It is amazing what can be achieved for eyes by homeopathy.

In this section I have assumed a correct diagnosis has been made, and I suggest homeopathic remedies which can help, either on their own or alongside conventional treatment. Most of the remedies should be given twice daily.

Injuries
Arnica Montana 30c when there is bruising from the injury.

Ledum Palustre 6c for a puncture wound of the eyeball, or the eyelids.

Symphytum 30c can produce a remarkable recovery from any blow in the region of the eye. It is particularly indicated for blows from blunt objects, such as the eye being hit by a door, or by your dog being kicked by a horse. It may also be used for blocked tear ducts, especially when this is the result of an injury.

Eyelid Problems
Entropion is the condition where the eyelids turn inwards and rub on the surface of the eye. It is painful, and can cause ulceration of the surface of the eye. Generally it is best corrected surgically.

Ectropion is where the eyelid turns out. It is generally less serious than entropion. However the eye is prone to infection, there can be discharges from the eye and the general appearance can be unpleasant. Please refer to the section on conjunctivitis below for remedies to treat these discharges.

Borax 6c helps mild cases of both these problems. Give one tablet twice weekly for three months.

Inflammation of the eyelids themselves is called *Blepharitis*. Inflammation of the inside lining of the eyelids is *Conjunctivitis*. Ulcers or infection may be present in both these conditions. For these problems I suggest:

Aconitum Napellus 30c when the lids are red and swollen, and the eyes are running. They may be painful and the dog may dislike bright light.

41

Acidum Nitricum 30c when there is ulceration of the lids. It is particularly useful for lesion involving the margins of the lids.

Apis Mellifica 6c when there is just a simple puffiness of the eyelids. Give one tablet twice a day for three days. It is also indicated in those cases where the conjunctiva becomes very swollen, and appears like a blister.

Euphrasia 6c when there are a lot of painful tears and the dog is continually blinking.

Graphites 6c when the skin of the eyelids is moist and sticky. The eyelids themselves may be stuck together by the discharges.

Hepar Sulphuris Calcareun 30c when there is a profuse watery discharge.

Mercurium Corrosivus 6c when infection is present and there is a green discharge.

Natrum Muriaticum 6c when there are profuse, painful tears and the lids are tightly closed.

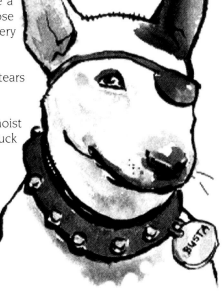

Symphytum 30c helps eyes to recover from injury.

Picricum Acidum 6c when the problems are longstanding and chronic. There is a lot of thick yellow discharge.

Pulsatilla 6c when there is infection with a creamy discharge.

Rhus Toxicodendron 6c when Apis Mellifica has not completely cleared the swelling. It also helps when eyes are red and sore.

Staphysagria 6c when the skin around the eye is also sore or inflamed (periorbital eczema). It is also very useful for treating swellings and tumours of the third eyelid. Homeopathic treatment may avoid surgical removal of the third eyelid.

Thuja 6c for warts and tumours on the eyelids. Surgical removal of these lumps may produce an uneven margin to the eyelid.

Tellurium 30c for eyelids which are thickened and scaly.

Urtica Urens 6c when an allergy is suspected.

Eyelashes
Ingrowing or misplaced eyelashes should be removed to prevent damage to the eye.

Borax 6c will help relieve the soreness.

Dry Eye

This is a condition where tears are not produced properly. The drying of the eye can lead to severe, irreversible damage to the eye, so a vet's advice and treatment with artificial tears are essential. There are surgical treatments which may help this problem.

Zincum Metallicum 30c twice daily, as well as using the artificial tears, can be given if appropriate conventional treatment or surgery is delayed. If there is an improvement, it may be better to continue to give homeopathic treatment rather than resort to surgery.

Chalazion

A chalazion is a small, painless nodule on the edge of the eyelid. Of itself it is not serious, but it can be unsightly.

Thuja Occidentalis 30c or Callarea Fluorica 30c twice daily for three days, then one twice a week, will remove it after a period of time.

Staphysagria 6c is also a useful remedy and is particularly useful if the eyelid is sore.

Styes

A stye is a painful round swelling on the inner edge of the eyelid. Usually it is infected. I suggest using:

Staphysagria 6c as the first remedy for this problem.

Hepar Sulphuris Calcareum 30c if the eye is very painful. Give the remedy every hour until the pain lessens.

Calcarea Fluorica 30c or Silicea 30c, twice weekly, for persistent cases which do not appear to respond to the other remedies. These remedies may take a some time to work.

Tear Ducts

The tear ducts, which drain the tears from the eye to the nose, can become blocked. This may be due to injury, infection, or the ducts may have not developed properly. This is more common in the snub-nosed breeds such as the bulldog and the pekingese.
    I suggest using:

Natrum Muriaticum 6c when there is infection in the duct. Very often pus can be expressed by pressing on the corner of the eye close to the nose.

Symphytum 30c if the problem has been caused by an injury, or poor development of the duct. The latter problem responds better in young dogs. It may take several weeks to improve. I recommend giving one tablet twice daily for three days, and then one tablet twice a week.

Eyeball Problems

The cornea is the clear surface of the eye and any problem usually produces pain, cloudiness of the cornea, and closing of the eye. Damage to the cornea may result from infection and inflammation. It may also result from rubbing by ingrowing eyelashes and other injuries. It is important that the cause of the damage is removed.

The normal healthy cornea is clear and does not contain blood vessels. Nearly always, damage to the cornea causes an ulceration of the cornea. This means that the outer, shiny, protective layer has been removed, and the underlying layers are eroded, producing pits of varying depths. In extreme cases the cornea may perforate, structures from inside the eye are forced into and through the hole, producing a swelling on the surface of the eye. This is called a keratocoele or staphyloma. The condition can also result from a bad puncture wound. This alarming condition responds well to homeopathy.

During the healing of severe damage, the cornea is invaded by blood vessels. These carry the nutrients needed for the healing process to the cornea. The blood vessels are clearly visible, and may even make a complete red circle around the lesion. The blood vessels also bring cells which create black pigment into the cornea. These cells can remain after healing is complete, and create a black opaque pigment layer over the cornea, impeding eyesight. I suggest giving:

Apis Mellificum 6c when a keratocoele is present. When used for the first few days, it will reduce the swelling. Then give **Mercurius Solubilis 6c** to promote the final healing.

Argentum Nitricum 6c when the eye is closed, red and painful. Give one tablet four times daily until the symptoms have gone.

Calcarea Carbonica 6c for a chronic indolent ulcer, often found in a fat animal. Give one tablet twice a day for three days, and then one twice a week. Usually these ulcers are very shallow, but involve a comparatively large area of the cornea. They can take a long time to heal completely.

Euphrasia 6c when the eye is very watery and very sensitive to light. The dog is continually blinking.

Kali Bichromicum 6c when there is a discharge of yellow 'ropy' mucus. It is of particular help in the overweight dog.

Ledum Palustre 6c for a simple puncture wound.

Mercurius Corrosivus 6c for a very deep ulcer. It is also useful if there is a green discharge.

Mercurius Solubilis 6c will help the healing process and, if given for a long period of time, reduces pigmentation of the cornea.

Inflammation of the structures within the eye is called ***uveitis***. When the whole eye is inflamed there is severe pain and the pupil is contracted. I advise using:

Aconitum Napellus 30c in the very early stages. Three doses, at hourly intervals, can be enough to relieve the pain.

Phosphorus 30c for cloudiness in the eye, and if the eyeball is becoming swollen.

Rhus Toxicodendron 30c will help to clear the inflammation. The eyelids may be swollen, and there may pus in the eye.

Cataract
Cataract is the name given to any opaque cloudiness of the lens. It can be recognised as a grey or white mass filling the whole of the pupil. It is frequently seen in the older dog. I advise using:

Calcarea Carbonica 6c for the overweight and idle dog.

Conium Maculatum 6c in the early stages, and when the problem is associated with old age.

Phosphorus 30c or Silicea 30c in longer standing cases. Give one tablet twice a day for three days and then one tablet twice a week.

Some forms of cataracts are associated with *Diabetes Mellitus* (sugar diabetes) and *chronic nephritis*. These may respond when the diseases are treated.

Glaucoma
This is a swelling of the eyeball. It is a very serious problem, and is difficult to treat. The pressure within the eye can become so great that the structures within the eye are destroyed, causing blindness.
  I suggest using:

Aconitum Napellus 30c given three times at hourly intervals, and in the very early stages, is helpful in relieving distress.

Apis Mellificum 6c can reduce the swelling.

Colocynthis 6c may be used to relieve the pain.

Phosphorus 30c is a very good longer term remedy, particularly when there is cloudiness in the eye.

The **retina** is the light-sensitive membrane at the back of the eye, inside the eyeball. All sight depends on this membrane receiving light and sending messages to the brain. It may be destroyed in cases of glaucoma.

Progressive Retinal Atrophy
Dogs also have a disease which gradually destroys the retina. It is called Progressive Retinal Atrophy, and is usually hereditary.

Phosphorus 30c is helpful in slowing, and sometimes stopping, retinal destruction. It cannot replace the retinal tissue which has already been destroyed. I give one tablet twice daily for three days and then continue giving one weekly.

female problems

Bitches of the smaller breeds generally come into season at approximately six monthly intervals. In the larger breeds the seasons may be less frequent, and the intervals between them may be as long as 12 or 15 months. Signs of being in season are swelling of, and bleeding from, the vulva. Also the bitch spends a lot more time licking and cleaning her vulva. These signs are more difficult to detect in small breeds.

The season lasts about three weeks. During this time the bitch is fertile, and is attractive to, and attracted by, male dogs. A normally obedient bitch may do everything in her power to escape and find a mate so, please, do make sure that your bitch is always secure. When she is in season, always exercise her on a lead and avoid any unplanned mating. There are too many unwanted puppies in this world as it is.

After the season has finished, all bitches, whether they are pregnant or not, go through the same hormone changes. Most of these changes take place during the nine weeks after the season. This is the period when a mated bitch would be pregnant. These hormone changes produce many of the female dog's problems. Conventionally the problems can be treated with hormones, or be prevented by spaying the bitch.

Spaying means removing the whole womb and the ovaries. However, this alters the metabolism, and many bitches put on weight in spite of dieting. In turn, excessive weight can cause heart or leg problems. Strict dieting can result in a hungry bitch who turns to stealing or raiding dustbins, an activity not popular with the neighbours!

Homeopathy can offer alternative treatments which avoid the drastic step of spaying your bitch.

Cystic Ovaries and Nymphomania

In this condition the follicles in the ovary which bear the eggs do not burst as they should. They remain in the ovary and continue to produce the hormones which bring about the bitch's season. The dog remains permanently in season, attractive to male dogs, and frequently there is a great deal of bleeding from the vulva. Conventional treatment is to spay the bitch or to use hormones. Spaying is the treatment of choice if the bitch is ill. Hormones can cause your dog to develop pyometra later in the cycle.

Homeopathy can offer further alternatives. I suggest you use:

Apis Mellifica 6c three times daily for five days is the first remedy to try. It is especially indicated for the indifferent, whining character. It is also useful if the vulva becomes excessively swollen. If the problem persists, try:

Cantharis 6c when the vulva is a very dark colour or painful.

Colocynthis 6c when the abdomen appears painful. Give one tablet twice daily for seven days. Stop the treatment if the pain is relieved earlier. This may also help if the bitch has become irritable and bad tempered.

Phosphorus 30c when the bitch is oversexed. She may continually seek a mate, or may behave in an unacceptable manner, such as riding furniture and people.

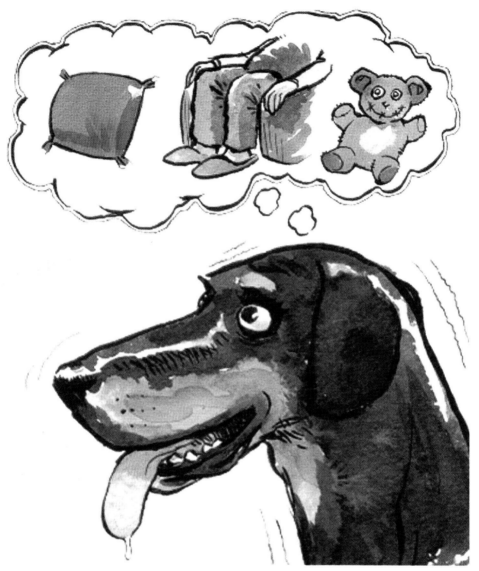

Your bitch may be looking for a mate, and behaving in an anti-social manner.

Tarentula Hispania 30c is also useful for the oversexed and hysterical bitch.

False or Phantom Pregnancy
All bitches, whether they are pregnant or not, go through the hormone changes of pregnancy. Most bitches are not affected by these changes but some, who are not pregnant, show all the signs and behaviour of pregnancy. About nine weeks after the season, or a little earlier, they may start making nests for their phantom puppies. The breast glands may become enlarged and even produce milk. Conventionally, the bitch is treated with hormones and you may be advised to have her spayed to prevent further problems. Spaying can itself produce problems, as described in the paragraph above, so there is every good reason to try homeopathy.

47

I suggest using:

Sepia 30c as one of the two main remedies to use to sort out these tangled-up female hormones. It is particularly useful in the bitch who may be bad-tempered, sulky, and who jealously guards her nest.

Pulsatilla 30c is the other main remedy for false pregnancy. It suits the bitch who is more gentle, affectionate and shy. There may be creamy discharge from the vulva.

Also consider using:

Bryonia Alba 6c to help when the breast glands are hot and swollen. It is particularly useful for the bitch who is reluctant to move. Do consider whether there is an infection in the glands. Please see the section on mastitis below.

Calcarea Carbonica 6c when the breast glands are hot and swollen with milk. It is useful for the fat and lethargic bitch.

Lachesis 30c when there is a great deal of bleeding. It is especially indicated for the jealous, suspicious bitch.

Urtica Urens 3x or a lower potency is useful for drying up milk. You must give this remedy in low potency. High potency may encourage milk flow.

Infection of the Breast Glands or Mastitis
Infections of the breast glands may occur in bitches which produce milk with a false pregnancy. Also, infections may occur in the pregnant bitch, both before or after whelping. Tumours of the glands can become infected. The appropriate antibiotics should be given. Homeopathy helps to achieve a complete cure. I suggest you use:

Apis Mellifica 30c when there is a great deal of painful swelling of the glands and the surrounding tissue. This is most common soon after whelping.

Belladonna 30c when the glands are hot and swollen. The bitch may be restless and excited.

Bryonia Alba 30c when the glands are very hard. The bitch may be constipated, and her legs may be stiff.

Hepar Sulphuris Calcareum 30c when the glands are very painful. There may be a thin, pussy discharge.

Phytolacca 6c when there are hard, painful lumps in the breast glands. The glands may have a blue colour and the bitch may be listless.

Urtica Urens 1m may be given to restore milk production as the infection subsides. This remedy must be given in high potency. Low potency may reduce milk flow.

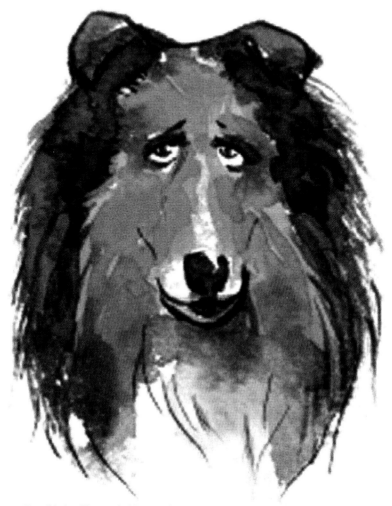

Your bitch will soon feel better after the appropriate remedy is given to her.

Tumours

Tumours of the breast gland, called mammary tumours, are quite common in the bitch. Some are cancerous and some are not. Surgical removal can be very successful. Spaying prevents mammary tumours developing in most bitches. Homeopathy can be very helpful in controlling mammary tumours, and may be indicated when there is a reason for not operating, such as extreme old age. Antibiotic treatment may also be used when the glands are infected.

I suggest giving:

Asterias Rubens 6c when a cancerous tumour has ulcerated.

Calcarea Fluorica 6c when the tumours are small and hard. It may be used in the early stages of the problem. Treatment needs to be continued over a long period. I recommend one tablet twice a day for five days, then one tablet twice a week. When

49

the tumour has become smaller, consider giving one tablet every fortnight to discourage it from growing again.

Conium Maculatum 30c can be given to the older bitch who may also be weak on her hind legs, and may tremble. I give one tablet twice a day for three days and then one weekly.

Hydrastis Canadensis 30c can be used for the cancerous tumour which has not ulcerated. The tumour is hard, with an irregular outline, and there may be a yellow discharge from the nipple.

Phosphorus 30c when there is an infection with a bloody discharge from the nipple. It is helpful to the thin, weak bitch.

Phytolacca 6c when the breast glands are hard and painful. There may be infection present, and the bitch is restless. It is is also a good remedy to give in the early stages of the problem as it can stop further development of the tumours.

Thuja Occidentalis 30c for vaginal polyps. These are tumours of the vagina which may be visible through the vulva. They are difficult to remove surgically.

Pyometra

This is a very serious, and potentially fatal, condition where the womb fills with fluid which may become infected. It usually occurs about 6–10 weeks after the bitch's season has ended. The bitch drinks a lot. She may vomit and there may be a discharge from the vulva. She may spend a lot of time licking her vulva. It is extremely serious if the bitch is vomiting and there is no discharge. She can die very quickly from the effects of the poisons developing in the womb, so diagnosis and treatment by your vet is essential.

There is no doubt that the best treatment is to remove the ovaries and the womb. This removes the cause of the problem. The bitch cannot come in season again, and she has no womb. Therefore the problem cannot recur. If the bitch is not spayed, it is almost certain that pyometra will develop again after her next season.

If for any reason surgery cannot be undertaken, homeopathy can be used to alleviate the problem. Best results are achieved when treatment is given in the early stages of the problem. I suggest:

Caulophyllum 30c when the purulent fluid, which may be chocolate coloured, is discharging from the vulva.

Pulsatilla Nigricans 30c when the discharge is creamy. The bitch may be shy and affectionate.

Sepia 30c is a major remedy which can sort out female hormones and womb problems. It is especially useful for the sulky, bad tempered bitch. The discharges may be yellow or green.

first aid

First aid should, literally, be first aid. It is the immediate help you can give your dog in an emergency. If your dog is seriously injured or collapses, then it must be in his best interests to seek a vet's help as quickly as possible. However, this section gives the homeopathic remedies you may want to use as first aid treatments.

Bites
Snake bites must be taken very seriously. Seek immediate help from a veterinary surgeon. It is most unlikely that you will have a suitable homeopathic remedy immediately available. For bites from other dogs or cats I suggest you give:

Arnica Montana 30c four times a day to relieve bruising and pain.

Hepar Sulphuris Calcareum 30c to prevent infection and to relieve pain.

Hypericum Perforatum 6c to relieve pain from nerves injured by the bite. It is particularly useful for damaged toes. Give one tablet every hour until the pain is relieved.

Collapse from Shock
Aconitum Napellus 30c to alleviate the pain and the immediate shock of the injury. I suggest giving one tablet every hour until the symptoms disappear.

Carbo Vegetabalis 30c is a most useful remedy for the collapsed dog who may appear to be dying.

Heat Stroke
This is not a common condition where dogs have the choice of sun or shade. Sadly, every year one sees dogs who have been left in a car in hot sunshine. Even with the windows open, a dog can suffer heat stroke. If you have to leave your dog in the car, please make sure it is in the shade. Better still, do not take your dog with you in hot weather if he has to be left in the car. He will be more comfortable, safe, well and happy in his own bed at home. However, if heat stroke does occur, I suggest using:

Belladonna 30c when the dog makes convulsive movements, is twitching or is excited.

Bryonia Alba 30c when symptoms are worse for trying to move.

Gelsemium Sempervirens 30c when there is prostration, drowsiness or trembling.

Sulphur 30c when the orifices, such as the mouth and eyes, are very red.

Insect Bites and Stings

Apis Mellifica 30c is indicated when there is intense painful swelling.

Cantharis 30c is useful for itching, burning vesicles. Vesicles are fluid-filled blisters which may be large, or small and numerous. They may appear as a rash.

Hypericum Perforatum 6c helps the sting which is painful but does not swell up.

Ledum Palustre 6c is indicated when there is bluish discolouration of the skin

Urtica Urens 30c helps when an itchy rash develops.

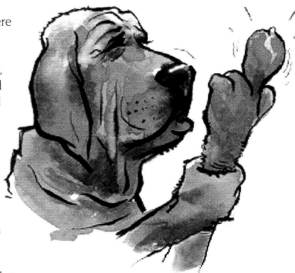

Arnica Montana 30c helps to relieve bruising and pain.

Road Accidents

The common injuries from road accidents are lacerated wounds, broken bones, shock and internal haemorrhage. Homeopathy can help wounds, shock and pain. Remedies are discussed in the section on wounds below. Internal haemorrhage, which may be mistaken for shock, needs immediate treatment by a veterinary surgeon. Therefore, after a road accident, do use homeopathy to relieve your dog's symptoms but take him to a vet as quickly as possible. Also, remember that your dog will be very frightened and in pain. He may try to bite you or other helpers as a purely instinctive action to defend himself. Approach him with care!

Arnica Montana 30c will help any injury or wound where there is bruising or pain.

Aconitum Napellus 30c will help the dog who collapses from shock, or is very frightened by his injury.

Rescue Remedy is extremely useful in treating or preventing shock. Simply give a few drops on the dog's tongue. Rescue Remedy is not a true homeopathic remedy; it is a combination of four Bach Flower remedies which are diluted in a similar way to homeopathic remedies. It is worth having the Remedy to hand all the time. It can be bought from some pharmacies, and from many health food shops.

Scalds and Burns

Aconitum Napellus 30c helps the dog that is frightened and in a state of shock.

Apis Mellificum 30c should be given when there is a great deal of pain and swelling.

Cantharis 30c is indicated when there is blistering of the skin.

52

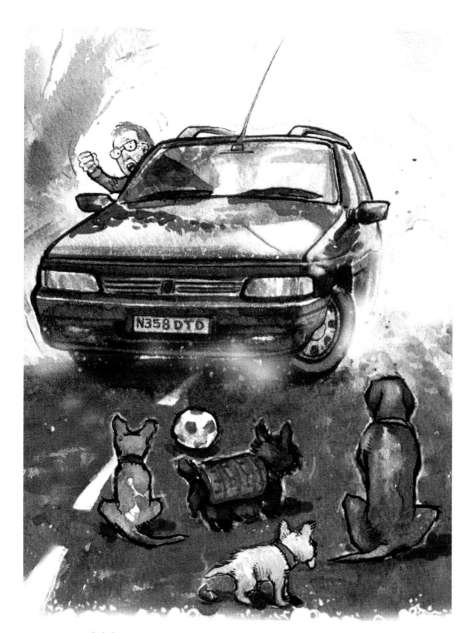

It is better to avoid accidents than to have to treat the after-effects.

Urtica Urens 30c may be given when the injury appears more as a rash.

Wounds

Homeopathy can help to relieve the pain and bruising from wounds. However, always consider the advisability of having a wound stitched up. Stitches are nearly always needed when a wound gapes open or when there is extensive bleeding. Pressure on the

53

wound, whether from a finger or a tight bandage, is a good first aid method of controlling serious bleeding, until help can be obtained from a vet.

Arnica Montana 30c every 15 minutes, for four doses, to reduce pain and bruising.

Calendula lotion or cream is very useful for scratches and abrasions which only affect the skin.

Hypericum Perforatum 30c will help when there is obvious intense pain. It is very useful for the lacerations that may be seen after a road accident, and in the treatment of crushed toes. Give one tablet every hour until the pain is relieved.

Ledum Palustre 30c should be given for puncture wounds, especially when the surrounding tissue is cold or blue. Foreign bodies such as thorns and hedgehog and porcupine quills should be removed. Porcupine quills are removed with a quick tug using a pair of pliers. If the tip breaks off, it should be removed by a vet as it can cause much damage by migrating through the dog's tissues.

Lachesis 30c may be indicated for the dog who has collapsed and is bleeding badly.

Phosphorus 30c may help small wounds which bleed a lot. Serious bleeding should be treated by a vet.

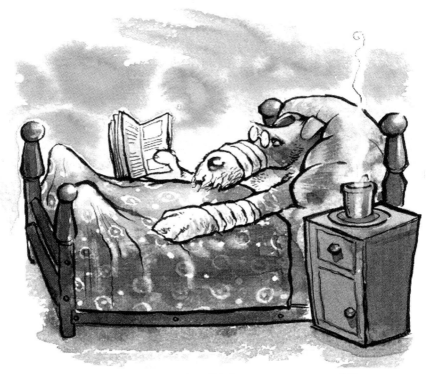

Lots of tender, loving care also will help your pet to recover quickly.

joints

Before treating your dog homeopathically for joint problems, do make sure that there is no other fundamental problem, such as a broken bone. Check with your vet. An X-ray will show fractures and also may highlight the changes associated with sprains and arthritis.

Sprains

The bones of joints are held together by ligaments. Put simply, each end of a ligament is attached to each bone, and holds them together. When your dog sprains a joint he becomes lame, and the joint becomes hot and swollen. He has in fact strained the capsule containing the joint, and the ligaments of the joint, damaging the places where they are attached to the bones.

Arnica Montana 30c is the first choice of remedy. It reduces the pain and swelling which is caused by the fluid that has developed around the injury. I give one tablet every 15 minutes, four times, and then one tablet four times a day for one to three days. When the swelling has gone completely, discontinue the tablets. Be prepared to use them again if the swelling returns.

Ruta Grav Graveolens 6c is given at the same time, to help the ligaments to heal. I suggest one tablet twice daily for three to five days.

Arthritis

When your dog has arthritis it means that he has an inflamed joint or joints. The joint is painful, may be hot and swollen and/or infected. The joint may be degenerating from age and wear and tear, or it may not have developed properly in the first place. Homeopathic treatment consists of looking carefully at the symptoms and finding the appropriate remedy. Again, if you can find a remedy which seems to fit the character of your dog, it is more likely to be successful.

The remedies listed below frequently alleviate true arthritis. Where conventional treatment is also needed, the homeopathic remedy often reduces the dosage of conventional painkiller or other medicine required. The remedies do not work well with the steroid group of drugs (cortisone).

If your dog is very stiff and in pain on leaving his bed in the morning, or after lying and resting during the day, and he gets better as he moves around, this indicates that the pain is worse after rest and is better for movement. If the pain increases as the day goes on, or during a walk, the pain is worse for movement. These characteristics direct us toward the two most important remedies for arthritis.

Rhus Toxicodendron 6c is indicated when the pain is worse for rest and better for movement. The pain may be worse in wet or damp conditions. It also suits the patient who is restless.

Bryonia Alba 6c is indicated when the pain is worse for exercise and better for rest. Your dog may prefer to remain still and cries out when moving.

Also think of:

Arnica Montana 30c if the pain is the result of a recent strain to an arthritic joint. It is particularly useful if there has been a recent injury to the joint.

Apis Mellifica 6c if there is a soft swelling of the joint. The pain is worse for heat and the patient is not interested in drinking. The joint is swollen.

Belladonna 30c when there is an acute infection, with a hot throbbing skin. It also suits the excitable dog.

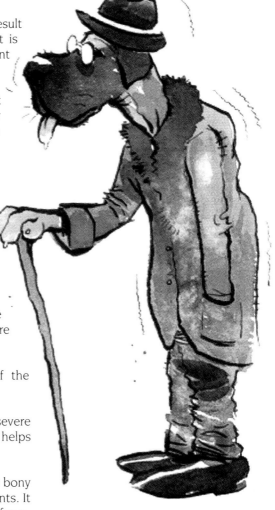

Calcarea Fluorica 30c is helpful in the later chronic stages, where there may be swelling of the joint, or of the surrounding bone. Your dog has enlarged joints. It is very good for treating conditions of the carpus (the knee). It is also indicated where there are cracking noises from the joints.

Caulophyllum 30c when the joints of the knees, ankles or toes are affected.

Causticum 30c is useful when there is severe pain, or the joints are deformed. It also helps muscular weakness and 'rheumatism'.

Hekla Lava 6c may be used to treat the bony lumps which arthritis produces around joints. It may be necessary to continue treatment for a long period of time. I usually recommend giving one tablet twice daily for three days and then one tablet once or twice a week.

An older dog often suffers from inflamed and painful joints.

Hepar Sulphuris Calcareum 30c is used when the joint is infected and painful.

Hypericum Perforatum 30c can be given when the joint has a puncture wound. Also, it is especially useful in painful wounds where nerve endings may be damaged, and in the treatment of crushed toes.

Ledum Palastrum 6c is also used when the joint has been penetrated by a sharp object, for example a thorn, producing a puncture wound. Do remember the wound may be infected. Ledum Palustre helps infected joints, but you may need to give an antibiotic prescribed by your vet.

Silicea 30c is indicated where there is a chronic infection of the joint, with little heat.

Hip Dysplasia
This is an inherited condition where the hip joint does not develop correctly. Good nutrition, not allowing the your dog to become overweight, and allowing only moderate exercise can slow the progress of the disease. It may appear in the very young dog, or it may not cause a problem until the dog is older. The 'ball and socket' of the joint is mis-shapen and there is excess movement between the bones, causing damage to the articulating surfaces. The result is arthritis and pain. Diagnosis can only be confirmed by X-ray. Conventional treatment is with drugs, to reduce the inflammation of the joint, with or without surgery. Surgery may modify the way the joint bears weight, or the joint can be removed entirely. The joint can be replaced with an artificial hip, or it may left to Nature to create a new fibrous joint.

All these treatments can be very successful, but they are drastic. They are painful and distressing for the dog. I have had many successful results from very simple homeopathic treatment:

Colocynthis 6c twice daily for three to five days, together with:

Rhus Toxicodendron 6c or Bryonia Alba 6c, depending on whether the dog is worse for rest or exercise. With both remedies, I dose twice daily for three days, and then gradually reduce the frequency. In most cases this produces a dramatic improvement. As with all arthritis cases, it is not a complete cure. Treatment needs to continue at a low, intermittent level. I usually recommend dosing once weekly to maintain the improvement.

Knee Cap
Some dogs suffer from a condition where the knee cap becomes displaced and the joint becomes locked. The hindleg becomes straight and stiff. When the knee cap returns to its normal position, the leg functions normally. This problem is more common in the very small breeds. Conventional treatment is to operate and try to construct ligaments which hold the knee cap in the correct place.

Homeopathy can also be very useful in treating this problem. I recommend giving:

Gelsemium Sempervirens 6c twice daily for three days. Then I reduce the dose to one tablet weekly until the problem disappears. If the problem recurs the treatment can be repeated.

At the same time, give:

Rhus Toxicodendron 6c if displacement is more common after rest, or

Bryonia Alba 6c if displacement is more common during or after exercise.

male problems

The Oversexed Dog
This is probably the most common problem associated with male dogs, particularly the adolescent dog. The behaviour can be very anti-social, whether it takes the form of aggression, unwanted sexual behaviour such as riding furniture or people, straying, or excessive territorial marking with urine, even inside the house. Conventional medical treatment is dosing with hormones, or the extreme measure of castration. Unfortunately, castration leads to a change of metabolism, and castrated dogs easily put on an excessive amount of weight. Dieting helps. However, many dogs seem to replace their sexual motivation with a desire for food, leading to new anti-social habits such as raiding dustbins or stealing food.

Homeopathic treatment of the oversexed dog involves careful consideration of the behaviour and character of the individual dog. It can remove the need to have the dog castrated, so it is definitely worthwhile to try homeopathy. If your dog is not castrated, please keep him under control so that he does not escape and mate. Already there are too many unwanted puppies in this world. I recommend using:

Chamomilla 6c for the young, excitable and snappy dog. He may whine. Also it is useful for the dog who salivates a lot.

Phosphorus 30c to reduce a dog's irresistible sexual desire. It is indicated for the excitable, nervous and fidgety dog.

Picricum Acidum 6c when the dog has prolonged and excessive erections.

Tarentula Hispanica 6c to reduce sexual desire. It is helpful for the hysterical, destructive dog, which may have an unreliable temperament.

Zincum Metallicum 6c will help the dog which has violent erections. The dog often appears lazy and stupid.

Lack of Sexual Drive
Most of us would consider this to be an blessing in the average pet dog! However, it is a problem for the dog who is intended for breeding. A lack of libido and impotence can be hereditary, so only consider treating dogs which have some other exceptionally good hereditary characteristics. Conventionally, hormone treatment is given, but homeopathy can also be very effective.

Agnus Castus 6c when the genitals are cold and relaxed. There may be a yellow discharge from the penis. It is helpful in the older dog.

Conium Maculatum 30c benefits the dog who is interested in the bitch but does not have an erection. It helps the older dog who may also be weak on his hind legs.

Lycopodium 30c will help the impotent dog who shows no interest in bitches.

Phosphoricum Acidum 6c helps the impotent younger dog.

Penis and Sheath Problems

When the penis or the sheath become infected there is an unpleasant discharge of pus from the sheath. Sometimes infection is associated with prolonged erections, and the penis may become strangulated. In these case the penis must be slid back into the sheath manually. Where the problem keeps recurring, the opening of the sheath may be too small, and will need to be enlarged surgically.

Homeopathic remedies include:

Aconitum Napellus 30c, given in the early stages, can help to relieve inflammation, pain and distress, particularly when the penis is erect.

Belladonna 30c is indicated when the tissues and skin are hot and red.

Hepar Sulphuris Calcareum 30c will help when the infection is deep in the sheath. Also, it is indicated for ulcers and pustules on the skin of the sheath.

Hydrastis Canadensis 30c when there is a thick, ropy and yellowish discharge.

Mercurius Solubilis 6c is useful in simple infections with a green discharge.

Mercurius Corrosivus 30c helps the more serious case, with a green discharge, that does not respond to the previous remedy.

Nitricum Acidum 30c is useful when there is ulceration on the penis, or around the opening of the sheath.

Pulsatilla 30c is indicated when there is a thick, yellow or creamy discharge from the penis or the sheath.

Thuja Occidentalis 6c may follow the other remedies to produce a more permanent cure. It is also useful for treating inflammation of the penis.

Prostate Problems

When a dog's prostate gland is enlarged it compresses the rectum, and makes it difficult for the dog to pass a motion. This is more common in older dogs. In younger dogs the gland may become inflamed or infected. Conventional treatment consists of hormone therapy for the enlarged gland, and antibiotics for infections.

Homeopathy can produce very good results. Prostate enlargement is an on-going problem in the older dog. Unfortunately, nothing makes old age go away! Treatment can be repeated when the symptoms recur, or it can be continual without having to worry about undesirable side effects. Frequency of dosing should be adapted to suit the individual dog.

I suggest using:

Ferrum Picricum 6c is the most valuable remedy for enlargement of the prostate in old dogs. I suggest one tablet twice daily for five days, and then one tablet twice weekly.

Hydrangea 3x when there is also a problem with stones forming in the urinary bladder.

Picricum Acidum 6c when the enlarged prostate is inflamed. It can also be used when the dog is oversexed.

Thuja Occidentalis 6c is of most use to the dog who has great difficulty in passing faeces. The enlarged prostate gland is pressing on the rectum, causing a partial obstruction. It can be used repeatedly, treating symptoms as they return.

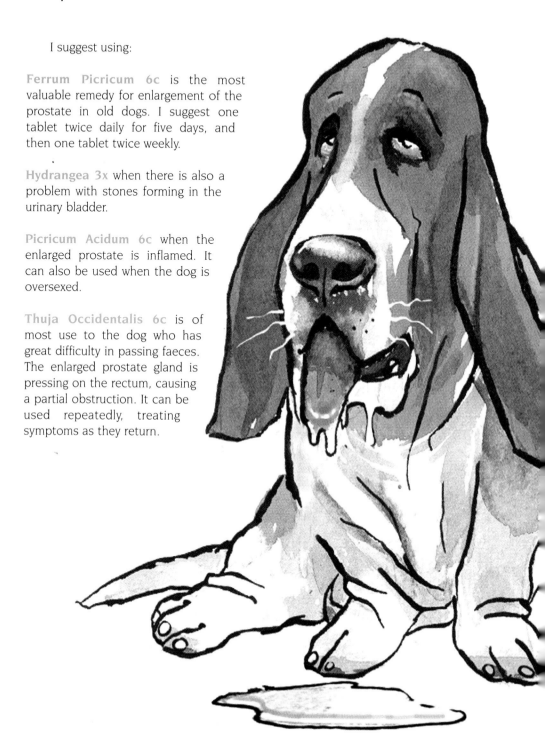

Excessive salivation can be helped with Camomilla 6c.

mouths

Lips

Inflammation is the main problem associated with lips. Homeopathy can be very helpful in curing problems. I recommend:

Borax 6c when there are ulcers on the lips which extend into the mouth. The ulcers may bleed. The surface of the lips may peel off easily. Typically, there is a large quantity of watery saliva that dribbles out over the lips. There may be vomiting, or a mucous and offensive diarrhoea, especially in young dogs.

Hepar Sulphuris Calcareum 30c when there are painful abscesses in the lips.

Mercuris Corrosivus 30c when there is an offensive slimy discharge of saliva.

Nitricum Acidum 30c is extremely helpful in curing inflammation in areas like this, where skin and the lining of orifices meet. It will also help the condition called Rodent Ulcer, which is a continually enlarging ulcer around the lips.

Rhus Toxicodendron 6c when there is a deep red discolouration, or small blisters on the lips.

Thuja Occidentalis 30c where there are tumours on the lips. Give one tablet twice a day for three days, then one weekly until the tumour disappears.

Mouth Problems

Most infections in the mouth produce offensive breath and excess saliva. You should remember that kidney disease, throat infections,

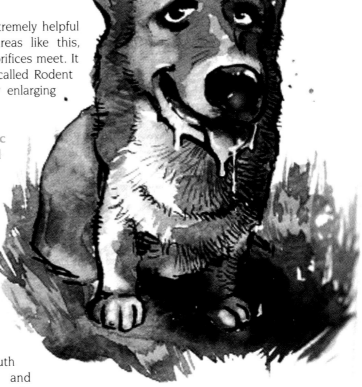

Try Mercuris Corrosivus 30c if there is a copious discharge of slimy saliva.

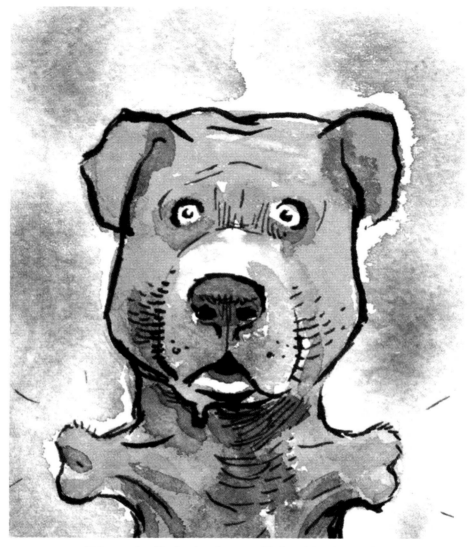
Make sure the offending item is removed before giving the remedy.

stomach disorders and tumours can also produce offensive breath. Homeopathic treatment may be used alone, or with antibiotics. I suggest giving:

Lachesis 30c may help when the whole mouth seems rotten and putrid.

Mercurius Corrosivus 30c is indicated where there is profuse production of slimy, smelly saliva. There may be bleeding from the gums. There may also be a bloody or offensive nasal discharge. Often the patient is excessively thirsty.

Rhus Toxicodendron 30c is helpful when spots and blisters appear. There may be dark red discolouration of the gums and lining of the mouth.

Phosphorus 30c when there is bleeding from the gums. The tongue is smooth and not thickly coated, although it may be red or white. To relieve the symptoms, the dog may seek to drink cold water.

Kali Chloricum 6c is indicated for the dog with kidney disease. There may be a lot of dribbling from the mouth. The dog may also have a greenish diarrhoea.

Blocked Salivary Duct (Ranula)
Your dog may develop a large blister-like swelling under the tongue. This is, in fact, a blocked duct from a salivary gland, called a Ranula. The fluid can be released by surgery. Often this produces a complete cure, but sometimes the Ranula keeps recurring. Homeopathy can be very helpful. I suggest giving:

Apis Mellificum 30c, three times daily for five to seven days to reduce the fluid.

Belladonna 30c if there is a painful inflammation. It also suits the excitable dog.

Mercurius Solubilis 6c when there is profuse salivation.

Thuja Occidentalis 30c if there is inflammation of the gums, or white blisters on the sides of the tongue.

Teeth
Veterinary dentistry has made remarkable progress in recent years, and a great deal can be done conventionally to improve your dog's teeth. Dogs rarely have cavities in their teeth, but they do suffer from a build-up of tartar. This enables bacteria to multiply and infect the gums and tooth sockets. Regular scaling can prevent this. Diseased teeth need to be treated by conventional dentistry.

Homeopathic treatment may be used to support dentistry. Infections can be treated in the same way as other infections of the mouth.

Arnica 30c reduces the bleeding, bruising and pain if your dog has to have teeth extracted.

Hekla Lava 6c may help when the jaw bones are eroded because of infected tooth sockets.

Fragaria 6c helps to prevent the build-up of tartar. I recommend giving three doses once a month.

Chamomilla 6c helps to relieve the pain and distress of erupting teeth. In a puppy this pain from teeth coming through the gums can cause all sorts of symptoms, from excessive chewing to fear and aggression.

Phytolacca 6c for the puppy whose mouth is very painful and may be bleeding. The tongue may be red and very sore. There may be a great deal of dribbling of stringy saliva.

Gums

Gum infections can be treated in the same way as other mouth infections. However, any associated teeth problems must be corrected.

Sometimes dogs develop a hard tumour on their gums called an E*pulis*. These are not malignant, but they can grow large enough to be a nuisance and also encourage infection. Conventional treatment is surgical removal.

This is often very successful, but the tumour can recur or it may become too large to be removed. These tumours respond very well to homeopathic treatment.

I recommend:

Calcarea Fluorica 30c, given twice weekly until the tumour decreases, as the remedy of choice for a fibrous tumour.

Calcarea Carbonica 30c is helpful in fat dogs. It is also useful when the problem occurs in young animals.

Hekla Lava 30c twice weekly for a bony tumour.

Throat Problems

Problems in the throat may involve the back of the mouth or the beginning of the gullet, the oesophagus. If there is damage to any of these areas, such as from a bone or a stick, make sure that the offending object is removed. You may have to seek the help of your vet, who will anaesthetise the dog to prevent it from biting.

Arnica Montana 30c, one tablet every 15 minutes and then four times a day can relieve bruising.

Infections of the throat may be local to the area or may be part of a more generalised disease. Homeopathy can be very useful, either by itself or alongside conventional treatment.

Aconitum Napellis 6c in the early stages of infection. Often this remedy alone produces a cure.

Belladonna 30c when the throat is red and puffy. Typically the dog feels hot and there is dilation of the pupils of the eyes.

Mercurius Solubilis 6c if ulcers are present.

Rhus Toxicodendron 6c when the throat is very red, and there is a lot of mucus.

nervous system

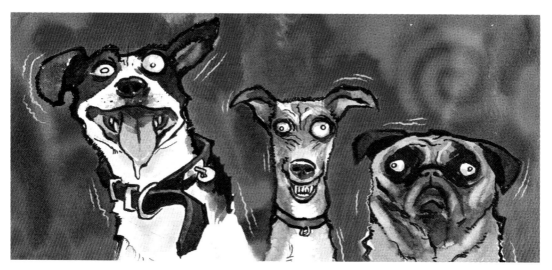

Homeopathy can help the excited, hysterical or depressed dog.

Convulsions are symptoms of a damaged brain. The damage may have been caused by an infection, such as distemper. The dog may have epilepsy, or a tumour in the brain.

Attacks often come on without warning. Sometimes, in epilepsy, the dog may appear restless or worried before an attack. When epilepsy occurs in the young dog under three years old it may be hereditary. Diagnosis of the cause of convulsions can be helped by your vet making an Electroencephalogram (ECG). Do make sure that your dog is suffering from convulsions, and not heart attacks.

Homeopathy can be very effective in treating convulsions. It is important to consider the dog's mental character when choosing a remedy. I suggest using:

Aconitum Napellus 30c when fear or fright produces the convulsions.

Belladonna 30c for relieving acute convulsions. Typically the pupils of the eyes are dilated and the dog will feel hot. The dog may vomit after the fit.

Chamomilla 30c for convulsions in puppies which may be associated with teething. The dog may be sensitive, irritable and thirsty.

Cina Maritima 30c for convulsions in puppies associated with roundworms, or with treatment for roundworms.

Cocculus 6c may be given once a week to help prevent the recurrence of convulsions.

Conium Maculatum 30c for the older dog who may show signs of old age, such as muscular weakness and trembling.

Gelsemium Sempervirens 30c for the dog who is also fearful.

Ignatia 30c when great excitement precipitates the convulsions. It is also indicated for the dog who grieving. He may be missing a previous home, a companion animal, or a member of the family.

Nux Vomica 30c for treating convulsions in the dog who is bad-tempered.

Plumbum Metallicum 6c when convulsions are associated with pain, which may lead to paralysis.

Twitching or Chorea
Involuntary twitching, and the continuous twitching condition called chorea, are usually the result of brain damage from an infection such as encephalitis. It is a common problem after your dog has had distemper. Please see the discussion of Nosodes (page 118–119)

Agaricus Muscarius 6c is a good remedy for chorea. It may also help the dog who chews himself obsessively.

Zincum Metallicum 6c helps the dog whose twitching is worse for being frightened.

Loss of Balance
This is often associated with brain injury, such as a stroke in the older dog. It may also be associated with an inner ear infection. Inner ear infections should be treated with the appropriate antibiotics. Homeopathy can help restore the sense of balance. I recommend using:

Belladonna 30c when there is an acute infection. The dog may feel hot, and the pupils of the eyes may be dilated.

Bryonia Alba 30c for the dog who continually falls forward.

Causticum 30c for the dog who continually falls, or circles to the right.

Conium Maculatum 30c for the older dog who may also show signs of muscular weakness. It can also help the dog who typically falls when shaking his head.

Drosera 6c when the dog falls to the left. It is also very helpful for the coughing dog.

Natrum Muriaticum 6c also helps the dog who falls to the left. Please see the section on Remedies for further indications of its use.

Rhus Toxicodendron 30c can be used for the dog who continually circles to the right.

Tarentula Hispania 30c is useful for the excited and hysterical dog.

noses

Nasal Discharges

Usually, in dogs, nasal discharges are caused by infections. They may begin as a clear discharge which, at a later stage, becomes purulent and bloodstained. Nose bleeds are not common in dogs, and are usually the result of injury. Sometimes a tumour in the nose may bleed. Other infections, such as distemper, can be the primary cause of nasal infections. Conventional medicine is to kill infections by using antibiotics. Tumours are difficult to remove.

Homeopathic remedies are chosen from observing the character of the discharge and the behaviour of the dog. I suggest using:

Arnica Montana 30c for any injury to the nose causing bruising or bleeding. I give one tablet every 15 minutes for four doses, then one tablet four times a day.

Aconitum Napellus 6c when it is thought that a sudden haemorrhage has been caused by shock or cold.

Arsenicum Album 30c when there is a watery discharge with scalding of the skin around the nostrils. Often the eyes run. The dog may drink small quantities of water frequently.

Calcarea Carbonica 6c for chronic discharges in the overweight dog. There may be bleeding, or the discharge may be yellow and offensive.

Cinchona Officinalis 6c to stop violent sneezing when there is very little discharge.

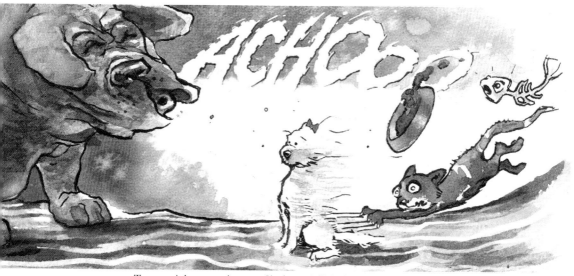

To stop violent sneezing, try Cinchona Officinalis 6c.

Ipecacuanha 30c in cases where there is bright-red bleeding. Frequently there is vomiting also.

Hepar Sulphuris Calcareum 30c when there is an offensive discharge, which may be worse for being in a cold wind. The nostrils may be sore.

Hydrastis Canadensis 30c when there is a thick, yellowish discharge. There may be ulceration of the nostrils.

Lachesis 30c when a nose bleed is accompanied by frequent sneezing.

Mercurius Solubilis 6c when there is a green discharge which may be bloodstained.

Nitricum Acidum 30c when there is ulceration and bleeding around the nostrils. There may be a greenish discharge, and your dog may sneeze a lot.

Phosphorus 30c when there is mild bleeding from the nose. This is usually from small blood vessels in the nasal lining.

Pulsatilla 30c when there is a creamy discharge. It suits the good tempered, affectionate dog.

Rhus Toxicodendron 6c helps cases which are worse in cold and wet weather. Also, symptoms may be worse after resting and sleeping.

Ruta Graveolens 6c is indication when there is spasmodic sneezing, and a lot of watery discharge from the nose.

Sepia 30c will help in cases of chronic discharge over long periods of time. Very often, there is an infection of the sinuses. I advise giving one table twice a day for three days and then one tablet twice a week.

Sulphur 6c is useful in cases when symptoms are worse for heat and there is an itchy, red skin.

Thuja Occidentalis 6c is indicated for tumours in the nose. It also acts when there is green, bloodstained pus.

Loss of Pigmentation
Sometimes dogs lose the black pigment from their nostrils, and the tip of the nose becomes a dull brown colour. This is not important to the dog's health, but it is to its good looks! It is also a disadvantage if the dog is to be taken to dog shows. I have had some success in treating this problem with:

Zincum Metallicum 6c, giving one tablet twice daily for three days and then one table twice a week. It may take several weeks before there is an improvement.

older dog

Like us, dogs can develop all sorts of problems as they grow old. Internal vital organs can deteriorate, and weakness and arthritis can reduce mobility.

Homeopathy can alleviate the symptoms of ageing and improve the quality of an old dog's life. Unfortunately, it is not a cure for old age. These problems are discussed here from the point of view of the older dog, but it is important to refer to the appropriate sections on the individual parts of the body.

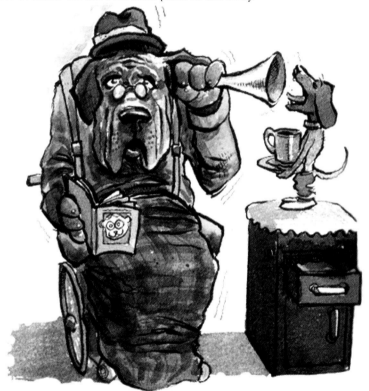

Like us, dogs can develop all sorts of problems as they grow old.

Ears

The commonest additional ear problem in older dogs is deafness. Of course, you have to be sure that your dog really is going deaf. 'Deafness' can be very useful when he does not want to hear! The dog who conveniently turns a deaf ear to your commands will continue to hear and to respond to noises that interest him, such as the sound of his dinner being prepared! Homeopathy can be very useful for genuine deafness. I recommend:

Causticum 30c to help the deaf dog who also has lot of wax in his ears.

Conium Maculatum 30c for the dog who generally is becoming weaker.

Lycopodium 30c when there is a yellow discharge from the ears. It is particularly indicated for the dog who may also have liver or kidney problems.

Phosphorus 30c for the dog who is lean. He may have lost weight from liver or kidney problems, and has a tendency to vomit.

Eyes

Cataracts and Retinal Atrophy are the most common eye problems of the older dog. A cataract shows as a bluish-white opacity developing in the normally dark pupil of the eye. It is common in dogs with chronic kidney disease. Retinal Atrophy means that the light-sensitive membrane at the back of the eye is disintegrating. This reduces the sensitivity of the eye to light so that the pupil, which remains dark, tends to be larger than normal. Your dog may not see as well in poor light or at dusk. Both these conditions are diagnosed easily by your vet. Either problem may cause your dog to go blind eventually, but homeopathy can be used to slow or arrest their progress.

Calcarea Fluorica 30c for the long-standing chronic cataract that is not responding to other treatments. Give one tablet twice a day for three days, then one tablet twice a week.

Conium Maculatum 30c for cataracts in the old dog who is becoming more frail.

Phosphorus 30c to stop further development of cataracts and Retinal Atrophy. It is especially useful in dogs with kidney and liver problems.

Heart

Dogs rarely have heart attacks similar to human heart attacks. However, as they grow older they frequently develop leaky valves. In addition, they may suffer from poor circulation which can affect every part of the body. These conditions may result in fluid collecting in the lungs and, particularly when exercising, the dog coughs. Also the dog may become lethargic and less inclined to move. Having said that, there are always the determined stalwarts who remain active against all the odds!

Dogs also develop irregularities of the heart beat. This may lead to a temporary shortage of blood to the brain and the dog collapses. This is similar to human fainting, and the dog recovers quickly. This is what happens when your dog has a 'heart attack'. It is not the same as human coronary heart disease.

Clearly, these serious conditions should be diagnosed and treated by your vet. There are very good conventional remedies for heart and circulatory diseases. Homeopathy can be used at the same time, often producing a spectacular relief of symptoms, and reducing the amount of conventional medication needed.

Bryonia Alba 30c to relieve the cough which is worse for exercise.

Cactus Grandiflorus 6c to assist the heart with leaking valves. Also it is indicated when blood pressure is low and circulation is poor. It is very useful in the early stages.

Carbo Vegetabilis 30c may resuscitate the collapsed dog who appears to be dying. It is also helpful in restoring normal breathing in the distressed dog. These attacks often occur in the evening.

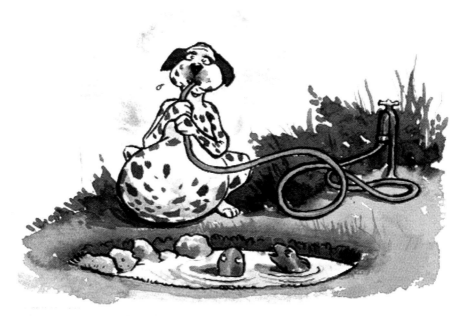

Excessive thirst may point to kidney problems.

Conium Maculatum 30c to relieve the cough which is worse for resting at night. It helps the dog who has become weak on his hind legs.

Convallaria Majalis 1x when the heartbeat is irregular.

Spongia Tosta 6c when breathing is gasping, and there is a chronic hoarse cough.

Lungs
Older dogs frequently lose the natural elasticity in their lungs, a condition called *emphysema*. This makes exhaling difficult. The dog may cough and appears short of breath.

Ledum Palastrum 6c may help this problem. I advise giving one tablet twice daily for five days and then one tablet daily until symptoms disappear. The treatment may be repeated when symptoms recur.

Kidney and Bladder
Chronic kidney disease (*chronic nephritis*) slowly destroys the kidney tissue so that symptoms occur in the older dog. These symptoms are commonly excess thirst, losing weight and developing cataracts in the eyes. In advanced cases, vomiting occurs because waste products accumulate in the body.

Treatment is difficult. Much can be achieved by a suitable diet, but help from your vet is essential. Homeopathy can relieve many of these symptoms. For the vomiting dog, the ease of administering remedies, and the fact that they can be absorbed through the lining of the mouth, are most useful. I described how you can crush the tablets to a powder in the chapter 1. I recommend:

Arsenicum Album 30c for the vomiting, dehydrated dog. (Please see the section about tummy troubles on page 89 for a description of dehydration.) The dog may drink excessively and the coat may be dry and dull.

Kali Chloricum 6c for the dog who dribbles excessively from the mouth. The dog may have ulcers in the mouth, or have a greenish diarrhoea.

Lycopodium 30c when there is a lot of sediment in the urine.

Natrum Muriaticum 6c when the dog is very thirsty, thin and losing weight.

Phosphorus 30c has a beneficial effect on the kidney tissue. It is particularly indicated when vomiting occurs a short time after eating, when stomach contents have become warm. It also helps cataracts in the eyes, as described above.

Incontinence of the Bladder
This is common in older dogs. The frequent, involuntary passing of urine may or may not be distressing for the dog. It is certainly distressing for the owner! Homeopathy can help relieve the symptoms, both for the dog and the owner.

Argentum Nitricum 6c for the elderly dog who is passing urine day and night. There may be very little urine, and this may be dark or bloody.

Causticum 30c when urine is expelled slowly, often during sleep.

Conium Maculatum 30c when there is constant dribbling of urine from the penis in the male dog. The dog may also show weakness of the hindquarters.

Hyoscyamus 30c when incontinence is accompanied by weakness and trembling of the muscles.

Pulsatilla 30c when urine is passed in sleep. It is more useful for the open-natured, affectionate bitch.

Sepia 30c can also be used when urine is passed in sleep. It is probably more effective for the irritable and indifferent bitch.

Legs
Arthritis and weakness are the two main leg problems in older dogs. For remedies for arthritis please refer to the section on Joint Problems (page 55). Homeopathy can help relieve leg weakness.

Conium Maculatum 30c is the remedy to consider trying first. It can give outstanding results in weakness of the hind legs. I recommend one tablet twice daily for three days, then one tablet twice a week.

Also consider giving:

Alumina 6c when the weakness seems generalised, and the dog appears partially paralysed.

Argentum Nitricum 6c when the weakness is accompanied by trembling.

Gelsemium Sempervirens 30c when weakness also affects the forelimbs. The dog may be easily tired by exercise.

Phosphorus 30c when weakness is accompanied by trembling and the legs suddenly give way.

Loss of Hair or Alopecia
This is common in the older dogs, and is often related to a problem with other organs. Please refer to the discussion of suitable remedies in the section on Skin Problems (page 85).

Thallium 6c is indicated for the dog with alopecia who is weak on his hind legs. It also helps when alopecia follows an acute or prolonged disease.

Restlessness
As dogs grow older their behaviour may change. They may be afraid of being left alone and are restless if left, particularly at night. This may lead to continuous barking. I believe that this behaviour is not just being naughty. It is because the older dog senses that he can no longer fend for himself, so becomes even more dependent on his owner. He is afraid of being left alone.

There are also old dogs who do not seem to know what they do want. When outdoors they want to come inside, and when indoors they want to go out! They seem confused. In fact, they are becoming mentally senile. Conventional medicine tries to relieve these symptoms with tranquillisers and sedatives, often making the dog spend lot of his time sleeping.

Homeopathy can relieve the symptoms without making the dog very sleepy. I recommend:

Argentum Nitricum 6c for the elderly dog who is anxious, apprehensive and seeks reassurance.

Arsenicum Album 30c for the dog who has also lost weight, and may have a dry, staring coat.

Conium Maculatum 30c for the dog who is confused. He is not sure where he wants to be. He needs company when he is alone, and wants to be alone when he has company!

Ignatia 30c may be given to the dog whose behaviour is contradictory. He may not like being alone. He may also suffer from some other sense of loss, such as death of a companion or moving house.

Lycopodium 30c for the dog who does not like to be alone. He may also have an ongoing kidney or liver problem.

Phosphorus 30c may help the dog who is also frightened by sudden noises and thunder.

pregnancy and birth

Problems Associated with Whelping

It is useful to treat your pregnant bitch with homeopathic remedies as a precaution against some common problems.

I recommend giving:

Arnica Montana 30c, one tablet twice weekly during the week before the puppies are due. Then give one tablet twice a day during the birth. This treatment will reduce damage and bruising to the birth canal. Also, giving Arnica before and after a Caesarean section will help the pain and bruising, and your bitch will recover more quickly.

Caulophyllum 30c once a fortnight during pregnancy. This helps to prevent complications and makes for an easier whelping. If, when whelping starts, the cervix does not open properly, give one tablet every 30 minutes for four doses. This may avoid the need for a Caesarean section.

Causticum 30c may help uterine inertia. The uterus becomes tired and normal labour contractions cease. Give one tablet every half hour until contractions return. If there is no progress within two hours, please seek help from your vet.

After whelping, I suggest:

Pulsatilla Nigricans 30c or Sepia 30c twice at 12 hour intervals to help the womb return to normal, and to help the expulsion of the afterbirths. Pulsatilla Nigricans is indicated for the shy, nervous and affectionate bitch. Sepia is the choice for the sulky and bad-tempered bitch.

Rejection of the Puppies

Some bitches do not want to suckle and mother their puppies. Frequently they appear afraid of them. I have found this problem is more common in pet bitches who are pampered members of the family. Homeopathy can be very helpful. I recommend:

Lachesis 30c for the bitch who is jealous and suspicious. The breast glands may have a bluish colour and there may be a discharge of dark red blood from the vulva.

Pulsatilla Nigricans 30c for the shy, affectionate bitch who may be afraid of her puppies. There may be a creamy coloured discharge from the vulva.

Sepia 30c for the bad-tempered and vicious bitch. She may attack her puppies. It is also useful for the bitch who is too protective of her pups and attacks you!

Failure to Produce Milk

Urtica Urens 1m given four times a day encourages milk production. Stop the treatment as soon as milk appears. This remedy must be given in very high potency. Low potency may reduce milk flow.

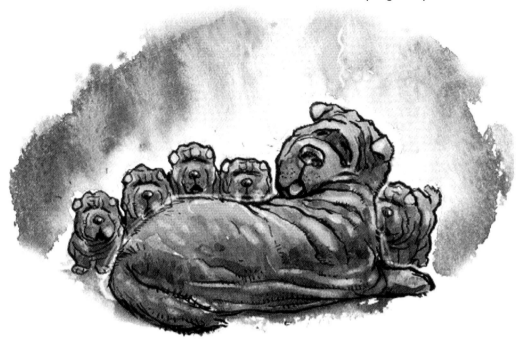

Encourage milk production with high potency doses of Urtica Urens.

Also consider:

Agnus Castus 6c for the bitch who may also have a transparent or yellowish discharge from the vulva.

Calcarea Carbonica 30c may help the bitch who is overweight and indolent.

Milk Fever or Eclampsia
This problem, which is caused by an upset in the calcium metabolism, may appear in the first fortnight after whelping. In the early stages the bitch may whimper, be nervous and restless. These symptoms get worse, leading to convulsions with rigid muscles. In these cases it is essential that the vet gives intravenous injections of calcium. The mother can die from this condition. Conventionally, calcium tablets are prescribed during pregnancy to prevent eclampsia.

　　Homeopathy can be useful, both to prevent and to cure eclampsia in the early stages. If the bitch is not able to swallow, crush the tablets between two teaspoons and place the powder in her mouth. The remedy will be absorbed through the lining of the mouth.

　　To prevent eclampsia I recommend giving:

Calcarea Phosphorica 30c one tablet weekly during the last four weeks of pregnancy, and one daily for seven days after whelping is completed.

In the early stages of eclampsia consider giving:

Belladonna 30c to help the bitch who is very excited and has violent convulsions.

Ignatia 30c to the bitch who is apprehensive, hysterical and trembling.

Zincum Metallicum 6c for the bitch who is lethargic. She may be very sensitive to noise. The breast glands may be painful and the nipples sore.

Please do remember that extra calcium is essential for the bitch with eclampsia and seek treatment and advice from your vet.

Infection of the Breast Glands or Mastitis
Infections may occur before or after whelping. They can also arise in cases of false pregnancy and in tumours. The appropriate antibiotics should be given. Homeopathy helps to achieve a complete cure.

Apis Mellifica 30c when there is a great deal of painful swelling of the glands and the surrounding tissue. This is most common soon after whelping.

Belladonna 30c when the glands are hot and swollen. The bitch may be restless and excited. The pupils of the eyes may be dilated, producing a staring, glazed appearance.

Bryonia Alba 30c when the glands are very hard. The bitch may be constipated, and the legs may be stiff.

Phytolacca 6c for hard, painful lumps in the breast glands. The glands may have a blue colour and the bitch may be listless.

Urtica Urens 1m to restore milk production as the infection subsides. This remedy must be given in high potency. Low potency may reduce milk flow.

Diarrhoea
Diarrhoea in unweaned puppies can be a serious problem. If any of the puppies are listless, please seek advice from your vet. In milder cases, the puppies remain active and continue to feed well. These puppies can be treated homeopathically. I recommend:

Aethusa Cyanpium 6c for the unweaned puppy who has a thin greenish diarrhoea containing undigested milk.

Further remedies are suggested in the section on Diarrhoea (page 36).

Weaning Problems
When the puppies are weaned, the mother may have too much milk and the breast glands become hard, swollen and painful. They may also become infected. Please see the sections on Mastitis above. I recommend:

Urtica Urens 3x to dry up the milk. This remedy must be given in low potency. High potency will encourage milk production.

Ignatia 30c for the bitch who is distressed because her puppies have been removed.

puppy problems

Most puppies who are fed a suitable nutritious diet grow up with no problems whatsoever. However, sometimes things go wrong. I do suggest that you have your new puppy checked over by your vet, who can tell you whether you have a normal, healthy pet. In this section I discuss those problems which you may want to treat homeopathically.

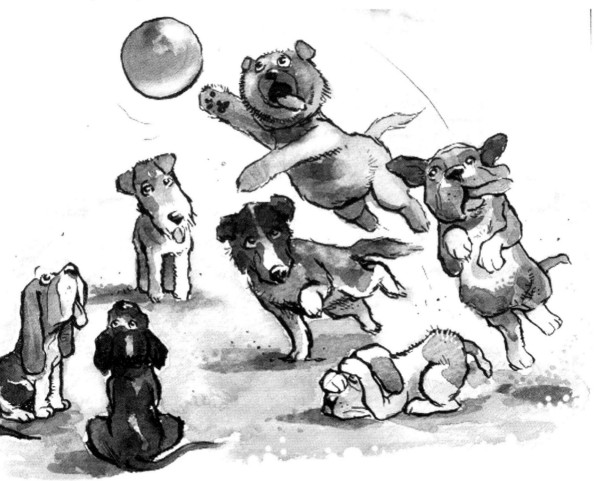

Exercise is fun, but a young pup should not overdo it!

Bones

These are problems mainly associated with the young growing bones. Rickets and problems from over-exercise are discussed in detail in the section on Bone Problems (page 29). However, homeopathy can help good bone development.

Calcarea Phosphorica 30c is ideal for encouraging healthy bone growth in young dogs. It is particularly indicated for the leaner, more active puppy. I recommend one dose daily for three days, and then one weekly for two to three months.

Calcareum Carbonica 30c to encourage healthy bone growth in the fatter, less active puppy.

Phosphoricum Acidum 30c to help developing bone in the rapidly growing dog. It is particularly useful when a young dog is lame after too much exercise, or has outgrown his strength.

Convulsions, Fits or Seizures

Fits in young puppies may be the result of an infection, such as distemper. The problem should be treated as discussed in the section on the Nervous System (page 65). When fits or seizures occur in puppies who have not been ill, you may dealing with a problem caused by the pain of teething or by a worm infestation.

I suggest:

Chamomilla 6c where the problem is associated with teething. The pain and distress is relieved and the subsequent fits may be prevented.

Cina Maritima 6c where the problem is associated with worms. This remedy is said to be able to destroy the worms themselves, as well as removing the symptoms of the worm infestation. However, I do recommend that you give conventional worm medicines to your puppy. Please remember to give the full course of treatment recommended by the manufacturer or the vet.

Teething

When your puppy is about four months old he will start to develop his permanent teeth. The premolars and the first molar teeth (cheek teeth) are the first to appear. The development of healthy teeth can be helped by homeopathic remedies. I recommend:

Calcarea Carbonica 6c when teething is delayed. It is indicated for the fatter, indolent puppy.

Calcarea Phosphorica 30c will also help in cases of delayed teething, but is indicated for the thinner, more active puppy. It may also be given once a week to encourage the development of strong, healthy teeth.

Chamomilla 6c to relieve the pain and distress produced by erupting teeth. In a puppy, the pain can cause all sorts of symptoms, from excessive chewing to fear and aggression.

Phytolacca 6c for the puppy whose mouth is very painful, and may be bleeding. The tongue may be red and very sore. There may be a great deal of dribbling of stringy saliva.

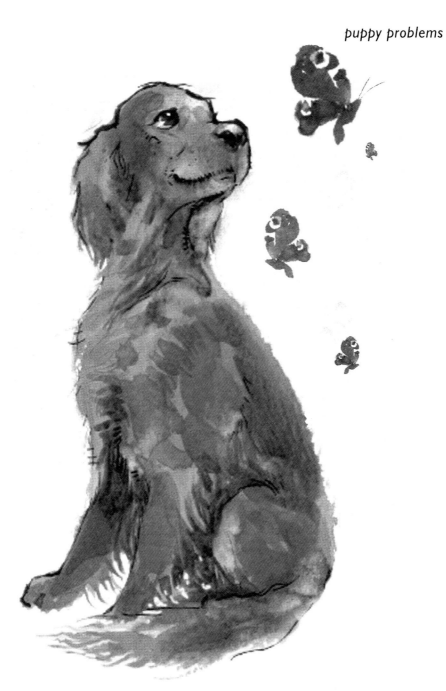

A happy, contented dog means a happy, contented owner.

Vaccination

Conventional vaccines are very, very good, and undesirable side effects are very rare. Homeopathically, dogs can be protected from infectious diseases by using the appropriate Nosode (Nosodes are described on page 118–119). The nosode, at the potency of 30c, is given twice daily for three days, and then one dose monthly for six months. A further dose is given every six months.

There is a practical snag in using homeopathy for vaccination. A vet can only sign a certificate of vaccination for a dog he has vaccinated. He cannot sign a certificate for a dog which you say has been given nosodes. These certificates are needed when your dog goes to boarding kennels, dog shows or when you are taking him from one country to another. In all these situations, only a certificate referring to a conventional vaccine will be accepted.

So, given the efficiency and safety of conventional vaccines, and the impossibility, at present, of satisfactory certification for homeopathic nosodes, I recommend that dogs should be vaccinated conventionally. Your vet will advise on a suitable course of vaccination for your dog.

Having said all this, there is still a place for homeopathic nosodes in the prevention of infectious diseases. They can be used where puppies are at risk from a disease and are too young to be vaccinated. They can be used in situations when a conventional vaccine cannot be used, such as when your dog is suspected of incubating the disease. They can be used to alleviate undesirable symptoms remaining after a disease has been cured. For example, distemper nosode given with other appropriate remedies may be used to help the dog who suffers from fits after recovering from distemper. However, you need to have an accurate diagnosis to treat these conditions. You are not treating the symptoms alone. Therefore, if you want to use the nosodes, I advise seeking the help of a vet who uses homeopathy.

Weaning
Homeopathy can help both the puppy and the mother at weaning time.

Ignatia 30c will relieve the grief and distress of both mother and puppies at weaning time and prevents them missing each other. It will also help the individual puppy who is distressed when he is removed from litter mates and is given a new home.

Urtica Urens 3x will help to suppress and dry up the mother's milk. This remedy must be given in low potency. High potency encourages milk production.

Phosphoricum Acidum 30c helps the puppy who has diarrhoea after weaning. The diarrhoea is involuntary and watery.

For other remedies for diarrhoea in weaned puppies please refer to pages 36–37.

Hiccoughs
Puppies develop hiccoughs very easily. They often occur after a meal has been eaten too quickly. Usually they disappear again very quickly and are not of any serious consequence.

Cinchona Deficinalis 6c is useful for the puppy who has frequent and persistent hiccoughs. Give one tablet every hour until the hiccoughs disappear.

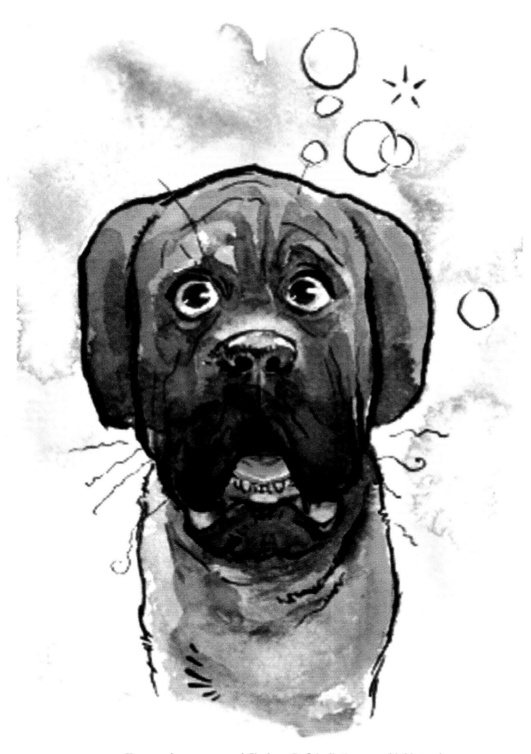

Your greedy pup may need Cinchona Deficinalis 6c to cure his hiccoughs.

skin problems

The skin is often described as the largest organ in the body, and it should always be thought of as an active and very important organ. It protects the body from external intrusions, can be used to expel poisons from the body, and has a vital function in regulating body temperature. Problems are caused by external invasions by parasites, fungi, bacteria and viruses, and by injury. They are also caused by disease problems within the body. Identification of the cause of a skin problem and its cure is notoriously difficult.

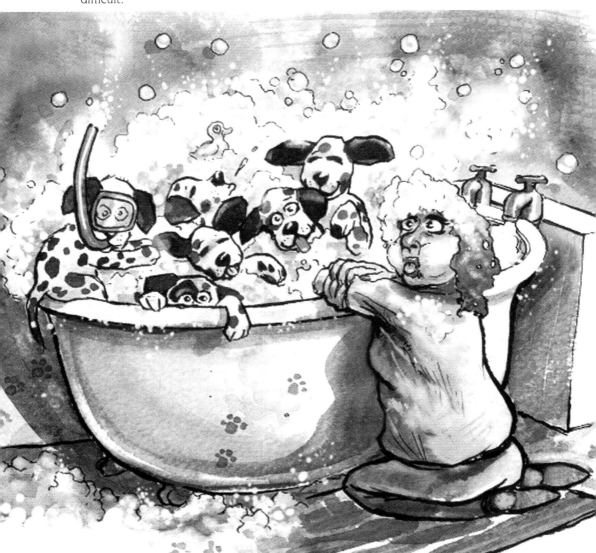

A medicated shampoo in the bath may help to clear up some skin complaints.

Therefore it is most important to obtain the best possible diagnosis of the cause of a skin problem from your vet. Infections, parasites or internal disease can then be given appropriate conventional treatment. This still leaves a large role for homeopathy. Where no accurate diagnosis can be made, homeopathy can produce a cure using remedies appropriate for the symptoms, or by using the dog's Constitutional Remedy. Of course, the best results are obtained if you are able to choose a remedy that fits the symptoms and the dog's constitution. Using the descriptions of remedies in this book can help you find the constitutional remedy. Also some skin diseases are caused by psychological upsets, such as fear or bereavement.

All these factors need to be carefully considered when selecting homeopathic remedies for skin problems. In this section I have listed suggested remedies for various symptoms, assuming that you are already giving a conventional treatment for the cause of the problem, where appropriate. Bathing your dog in the correct medicated

An allergy may bring your dog out in a rash.

shampoo can help enormously. As an added bonus, he is more pleasant to live with! Using steroids to alleviate skin diseases does not cure a problem, and prevents homeopathic remedies from working. In my opinion, these powerful steroids should only be used in acute cases, for a short time, to stop the dog from biting or scratching himself to pieces. They do not cure the problems. If they are to be used for long periods, they are likely to have undesirable side effects.

Sulphur 30c is the basic remedy to help skin problems. It encourages the development of healthy skin. It is especially indicated when the skin is hot and itchy. A rash may also be present. This is a very good general remedy which may be used alone, or to enhance the action of other remedies.

Allergies
Allergic conditions in the skin may be due to localised contact with a substance or creature to which your dog is sensitive, such as certain grasses or fleas. Alternatively, your dog may be allergic to substances which are not in direct contact with the skin, such as certain foods. Conventional treatment is to prevent further contact with the offending substance, and to give antihistamines or steroids to remove the symptoms. Homeopathy can be very helpful in removing the symptoms. Also, it may be used to desensitise the dog by giving the offending substance (allergen) in homeopathic doses. The allergen is made into a homeopathic remedy by diluting it. This is described earlier in this book when discussing remedies and potencies (see page 7). Sometimes the remedy may be available already, the obvious one being Pulex Irritans which is derived from fleas.

To treat allergies homeopathically I recommend:

Apis Mellifica 30c when there are large swollen areas of skin, which may be painful.

Astacus Fluiviatilis 6c when a rash covers the whole body.

Chamomilla 6c for skin rashes in puppies who are teething.

Pulex Irritans 30c when there are sore spots all over. It is especially indicated when the allergy is caused by fleas.

Pulsatilla 30c when lesions appear after rich food has been eaten. When appropriate, the diet should made less rich. Usually this means that the fat or protein content, or both, must be reduced. Chocolates and hamburgers are off the menu!

Urtica Urens 6c is the main remedy for urticarial swellings. These are red, blotchy lesions which look like nettle rash.

Bends of Limbs
Frequently quite severe skin lesions develop in the bends of the limbs, at the elbows, the knees or the stifle joints. There are specific remedies which can help.

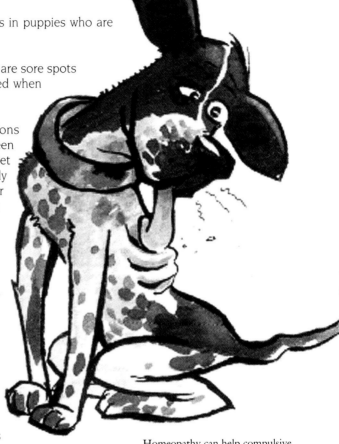

Homeopathy can help compulsive lickers...

Aethusa Cynapium 6c when the skin is cold, and clammy with sweat. There may be intense itching, and continual licking by the dog.

Ammonium Carbonicum 6c when there is intense itching and a scarlet rash or blisters are present.

Graphites 6c when there is a sticky exudate. Other parts of the skin may be hard and dry.

Kali Arsenicum 6c when the skin is dry and scaly. There may be intense itching, and cracks in the skin.

Lycopodium 30c when the dog also has a liver or kidney problem. It also helps when the skin has an offensive smell, and there is violent itching. The dog may be going grey at an earlier age than is normal.

Natrum Muriaticum 30c for the dog whose skin is greasy. The skin may be itchy and blotchy.

Sepia 30c when there are isolated, itchy, circular lesions which are not relieved by scratching. It may be especially helpful to the bitch who has recently whelped.

Blackened Skin
Blackened skin can be very unsightly. It is difficult to treat. I believe homeopathy is more likely to cure this problem and suggest:

Berberis Vulgaris 6c for a localised black lesion which remains after a problem, such as a wound or eczema, has been cured.

Kali Arsenicum 6c when the skin is itchy and thickened.

Sepia 30c when there is more generalised loss of hair. It is useful after mange has been cured. It may be particularly helpful to bitches after whelping, and to dogs who appear to feel the cold.

Cracked Skin
Graphites 6c is useful where the crack is moist and oozing.

Petroleum 6c when the skin is dry and cracked, and may also be red and inflamed.

Hair Loss or Alopecia
True alopecia is usually associated with an internal problem. The hair is lost in patches and bald areas appear, usually on the sides or lower back. The skin may become completely hairless and black. Homeopathic remedies which may help are:

Alumina 30c when there is intolerable itching which is worse for heat. The skin may be cracked.

Arsenicum Album 30c when there is scratching which is worse for being cold. The skin may be dry and rough or scaly.

... and chewers.

Kali Arsenicum 6c encourages hair growth.

Lycopodium 30c when there is a liver or kidney problem. There may be early greying of the hair, particularly around the muzzle, and the dog may be jaundiced. When a dog has jaundice the whites of his eyes and sometimes his gums and skin become yellow. Usually, a jaundiced dog is seriously ill, and should have treatment from your vet.

Natrum Muriaticum 30c for the dog whose skin is greasy. It suits the thin, thirsty dog.

Sepia 30c for bitches who lose hair after whelping. It is also helpful if the hair loss occurs about nine weeks after a season, the time at which a pregnant bitch would whelp. Hair loss in the non-pregnant bitch at this time may indicate that she is prone to the condition of pyometra. (Please see the section on female problems on pages 46–50.)

Thallium 6c when the alopecia follows an acute or prolonged illness. I recommend giving one tablet twice a day for three days and then one weekly. Treatment may be needed for several months.

Ustilago Maydis 6c may help when there are small pustules in the skin.

Hard and Thickened Skin

Calcarea Fluorica 30c may help localised, very hard areas of skin, and the condition known as a *granuloma*. This is a localised infection, producing a thickened area of skin. The dog continually licks the area, making the problem worse. In some cases the solution may be to remove the affected skin surgically.

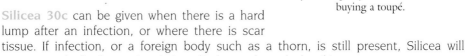

Try homeopathy for baldness before buying a toupé.

Silicea 30c can be given when there is a hard lump after an infection, or where there is scar tissue. If infection, or a foreign body such as a thorn, is still present, Silicea will encourage the body to reject it in a discharge through the skin.

Thuja Occidentalis 6c is useful when the thickening is more clearly defined, and may appear like a tumour or wart.

Sebaceous Cysts

Sebaceous cysts are swellings within the tissue of the skin, caused when a sebaceous gland becomes blocked. (Sebaceous glands produce the oily substance, called sebum, which keeps the skin moist and supple.) The gland continues to secrete sebum and blows up like a balloon.

In some cases, the pressure which builds up in the gland destroys the glandular tissue. Then the swelling does not get any larger, and there is no further problem. However, the cyst can become infected and burst. The cyst can also burst if the gland does not stop secreting sebum.

You need to be sure that you are dealing with a sebaceous cyst and not a tumour. Sebaceous cysts are contained entirely within the skin and, by picking up a fold of skin, you can pick up the cyst. Usually they are smooth and slightly soft. Tumours are harder and may have rough edges. If in doubt, please ask your vet for a diagnosis.

The burst glands never heal and have to be removed surgically. Also, surgical removal is the conventional treatment for the swollen gland which has not burst. Surgery may not be a desirable procedure, for example, in the elderly dog, or where a large number of cysts keep appearing. Homeopathy can help the problems.

Conium Maculatum 6c I recommend one tablet twice daily for five days, and then one tablet twice weekly until the cysts disappear, which may take several weeks.

Itching
Homeopathic remedies can help the dog who is continually scratching. They should be chosen according to the symptoms and, wherever possible, also relate to the dog's constitution and state of mind. I suggest using:

Alumina 30c when there is intolerable itching which is worse for heat. The skin may be dry and cracked, and the dog scratches until the skin bleeds.

Agaricus Muscarius 6c when damage and eczema are caused by hysterical chewing. It may also help when there are small, hot, hard areas of thickened skin, appearing like chilblains.

Ammonium Carbonicum 6c when there is violent itching and a scarlet rash, or the skin comes up in blisters.

Arsenicum Album 30c when the skin is scaly, dry and rough. Scratching is worse when the dog is cold. The coat may be harsh and dry.

Calcarea Carbonica 30c for unhealthy looking skin in the overweight dog. Scratching is worse when the dog is warm.

Cantharis 6c when there are blister-like lesions (vesicles) with intense irritation.

Carbo Vegetabalis 30c for the dog whose skin is cold. Irritation can be intense, and the skin may bleed easily. Also it can help cold, damp and smelly lesions between the toes.

Cinchona Officinalis 6c is indicated when the skin is very sensitive to being touched.

Hypericum Perforatum 6c when the irritation is the result of a puncture wound. It may also help the intense irritation from eczema of the feet. There may be hysterical chewing and biting of the affected places.

Ledum Palustre 6c for puncture wounds, particularly if the area feels cold. It helps irritations of the face.

Lycopodium 30c when there are swellings beneath the skin. The skin may crack and be thickened, and there may be an offensive smell. It may also help with eczema of the feet. Symptoms are worse when the dog gets hot. It is helpful to the dog who also has a liver or kidney problem.

Mercurius Solubilis 30c for vesicles or pustules, and the skin is always moist.

Mezerium 6c is useful when the lesions are mainly on the head. Small blisters may develop and burst to form ulcers, with a red area around them. The scabs which develop may run with pus. It often helps the condition known as Acute Moist Eczema. This is a very painful wet area of raw skin, which appears very suddenly. The hair may matt and stick over the surface of the lesion.

Natrum Muriaticum 6c may given to the dog whose skin is greasy. It may help lesions on top of the head and behind the ears. It suits the thin, thirsty dog.

Psorinum 200c Give one daily for three days for the dog with a dry, dirty looking coat and an offensive smell. This remedy can be particularly effective after an initial course of sulphur. It may take seven to ten days to work after the course of treatment is finished.

Rhus Toxicodendron 30c for skin which is red and swollen. Small blisters may be present. Symptoms are better for heat, dry weather and movement.

Staphysagria 6c for irritations and sores around the eyes. The dog may go completely bald and have sore rings around the eyes (periorbital eczema).

Sulphur 30c is particularly useful when the skin is red and itchy, and the symptoms are worse for heat. It will often enhance the action of the other remedies.

Tellurium 30c when the skin is thickened and scaly.

Urtica Urens 6c when there are red blotches or weals in the skin.

Toe Cysts and Grass Seeds
These are often called *interdigital cysts*. The dog licks between his toes frequently, and a small, hard swelling develops which may become filled with blood-stained fluid. A similar problem can be caused by a grass seed penetrating the skin between the toes. Grass seeds must be removed. If left in the foot, they migrate up the leg, producing a series of blisters and ulcers.

Graphites 6c may help the soft cyst which is filled with blood-stained fluid. The skin may be cracked and oozing.

Hepar Sulphuris Calcareum 30c helps in the early painful stages. If pus has formed the 6c potency will help to promote drainage.

Silicea 30c can be used for a longstanding problem where the cyst may be very hard. It also helps to reject grass seeds, or other foreign bodies such as thorns, and the tips of porcupine quills, from the toes. It relieves discharging places which do not heal.

tummy problems

Vomiting

Occasional vomiting is a natural activity to a dog. It is a means of getting rid of unwanted stomach contents which may be causing discomfort. Having said that, a dog will frequently eat his vomit, which is quite repulsive to us but perfectly normal to him!

Dehydration

Persistent vomiting, particularly if accompanied by diarrhoea, can be extremely serious. Your dog can quickly become dehydrated because he has lost so much fluid. Often, you can detect dehydration in your dog by gently pinching his skin into a fold. In the healthy dog, as soon as you let the skin go, it immediately slips back into shape and the fold disappears. In the dehydrated dog the fold may take several seconds to disappear. A young puppy can die from persistent vomiting and dehydration in as little as two hours.

Your dog may have a serious, acute infection, or he may have an obstruction in his gullet or his intestines. He may have some other illness such as kidney disease. Therefore, if your dog is persistently vomiting, please seek a diagnosis from your vet. He may also bring the vomiting under control, and correct dehydration with intravenous injections. In the meantime, do not give your dog anything to eat or drink. It will aggravate the vomiting and do more harm than good.

Homeopathy can be used in the less immediately serious cases, and also to support conventional treatment. It may be more practical to crush pills between two teaspoons and give them as a powder. Then the remedy can be absorbed through the membranes of the mouth, and there is no risk of it being vomited up.

Apis Mellifica 6c when your dog vomits but has a comparatively dry mouth. Stools may be watery and brown.

Arsenicum Album 30c when the mouth is ulcerated and dry. Usually there is simultaneous diarrhoea. The vomit may be bloodstained, or contain whole blood. Typically the dog is restless.

Berberis Vulgaris 6c when the dog is yellow and jaundiced because of a liver problem. The whites of the eyes and, sometimes, the gums appear yellow. Please consult your vet if your dog has jaundice. It is a very serious problem.

Occasional vomiting is quite natural, but do check with the vet if it becomes persistent.

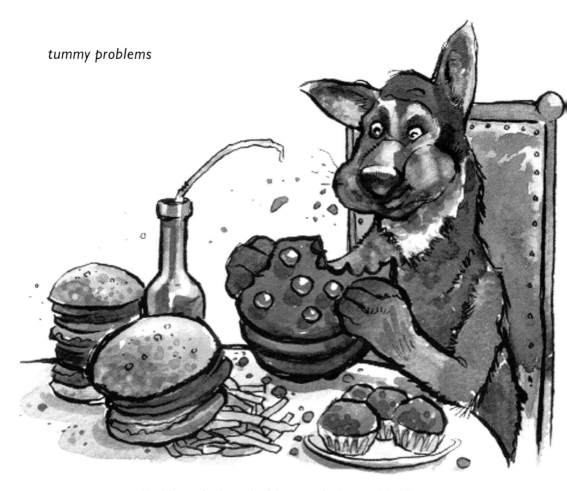

Vomiting can be the result of the wrong food or too rich a diet.

Carbo Vegetabilis 30c for the dog who brings up offensive wind.

Ipecacuanha 30c when there is frequent, slimy vomit, with a great deal of retching and distress. There may also be blood in the vomit.

Lycopodium 30c when the abdomen appears full and bloated. The upper abdomen may be tender, indicating liver disease. It is also useful when the abdomen is full of fluid (dropsy) as a result of chronic liver disease.

Mercurius Corrosivus 30c when there is great thirst with a constant cycle of drinking and vomiting. In these cases, water should be withheld until the vomiting is under control. This is because your dog actually vomits more fluid than he drinks.

Nux Vomica 6c when there is vomiting after rich food. Your dog may have stolen the Sunday joint! Stools are usually hard.

Pulsatilla Nigricans 6c is indicated in similar cases, where the food has been fatty.

Phosphorus 30c when vomiting occurs soon after eating or drinking. Usually sufficient time elapses for the food to become warm in the stomach. The gums may have ulcers, and stools may be pale. It is also helpful when kidney failure is the cause of the vomiting.

Travel Sickness

Travel sickness can be very distressing to dogs. Many dogs do not actually vomit, but they dribble copious amounts of saliva, look miserable and really are very unhappy. Then, of course, there is the dog who is actually sick, which is probably more distressing for the owner.

Conventional treatment is to give pills before the journey. These should be those designed for dogs, not humans. However, conventional treatments often make the dog sleepy, so he does not enjoy his day out. Homeopathy can work brilliantly. I recommend:

Cocculus 6c and Petroleum 6c together. Give one tablet of each remedy twice a day for three days. Then I advise giving one of each tablet about half an hour before a journey.

Diesel Smoke 6c may helpful when the vehicle has a diesel engine.

Often, after a period of time, and a number of journeys without being sick, the dog is cured.

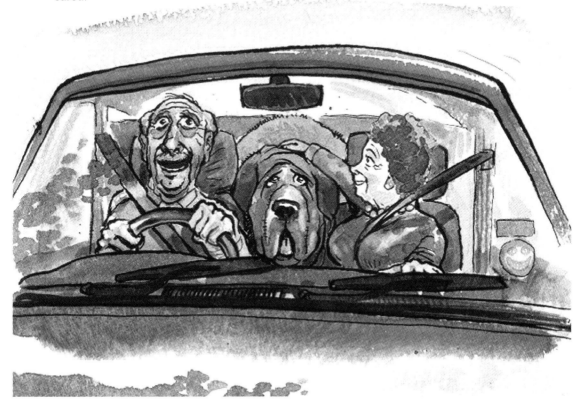

Prevent travel sickness with Cocculus 6c and Petroleum 6c and have a good day out.

tumours and warts

Tumours, warts and cancer can occur at any age, but are more common in the older dog. Conventional treatment usually involves surgery. The tumour is cut out. If the tumour is removed completely, before a cancerous tumour has spread, the cure can be complete. Chemotherapy and radiotherapy are also available and can be very successful in curing or producing remissions from cancer.

Homeopathy can also produce remissions and cures for cancer. I do not suggest that it is more successful than conventional treatment, but it may well be a more suitable treatment for tumours, warts and cancer where surgery is not possible. Many of these conditions can be treated with the same or similar remedies.

Below is a list of remedies to consider in the treatment of tumours. I have also discussed individual tumours in the relevant sections in this book. When a medical name is given to a tumour or other structure, you will find an explanation of the name at the end of this section. When there is a choice of remedy, please remember to try to fit the remedy to the dog's constitutional symptoms, and any other symptoms he may have.

I suggest using:

Asterias Rubens 6c for cancerous mammary tumours when there is ulceration of the skin. It is also helpful when there has been a cancerous spread from a tumour to the the regional lymph node or 'gland', such as the axillary and inguineal lymph nodes.

Calcarea Carbonica 30c for warts and polyps, particularly those on the young, fat and indolent dog.

Calcarea Fluorica for mammary tumours which are very hard. It is also useful for treating epulis.

Carcinosin 30c for tumours arising in epithelial tissue, such as anal adenomas and mammary tumours. Carcinosin should be given together with the appropriate remedy for the dog and his tumour.

Conium Maculatum 30c for tumours in the older dog. It should be considered for anal adenomas, mammary tumours which may be relatively soft, and tumours in the lymph nodes.

Ferrum Picricum 6c when large numbers of small warts appear in a small area. It is of particular use in treating warts on the feet.

Hydrastis Canadensis 6c may be given to relieve pain in cancerous states. It is also useful in treating hard, irregular tumours.

Ledum Palustre 6c when anal adenomas have deep cracks and fissures in them. It also helps the extensive, infected swellings around the anus, which occur most commonly in German Shepherd dogs.

Phosphorus 30c can be very useful for polyps in the nose, which tend to bleed. It is also useful for mammary tumours when the nipple is discharging pus.

Phytolacca 6c for hard tumours of the breast glands. The glands may also be infected and painful.

Thuja 30c is given to treat anal adenomas, lipomas, warts and polyps, whether internal or external.

Explanation of Terms

Anal Adenomas are tumours of the glandular tissue surrounding the anus. They occur in male dogs.

Epithelial tissue is the lining tissue found in all organs and glands. For example, it includes the lining of the mouth, mammary glands and the skin.

An *epulis* is a hard tumour on the gum. It is not malignant, but can grow large enough to be a nuisance.

Lymph nodes are the regional glands through which fluid drains from the relevant area of the body. They act as a filter, so cancer commonly spreads to them. The axillary gland is in the armpit and the inguinal gland is in the groin.

A *polyp* is a tumour arising on the surface of a tissue. It is usually pedunculated, that is, hangs from a narrow neck.

Anal tumours are tumours in the area around the anus. They start as quite small, hard swellings, but can grow together to become large, infected and smelly malignant masses. You will find them in the section on Anal Problems (page 22).

Some breeds seem to be more prone to tumours and warts than others.

urinary system

Kidneys

N*ephritis*, which means inflammation of the kidneys, is most commonly caused by infection. These days, your dog should be vaccinated against the most common infection, which is caused by the bacterium *Leptospira canicola*. The vaccination is a part of the routine inoculations your dog receives, together with distemper and parvovirus vaccines. Nevertheless, nephritis is still common.

Chronic nephritis occurs more frequently in older dogs. The infection gradually destroys the kidney tissue, and the kidneys cannot remove poisonous waste products from the body. The dog becomes thirsty, loses weight, and finally starts vomiting and becomes unconscious. The accumulating poisons in his body may cause convulsions. The problem should not be confused with *Diabetes Mellitus*, which can produce very similar symptoms. Your vet can confirm which problem your dog has by testing blood and urine samples.

In acute infections the symptoms are very similar, but may appear suddenly. Usually your dog will have a high temperature. The area over the kidneys in the middle of his back may be very painful. These infections come to the kidneys through the blood stream, and cause severe damage to the kidney tissue.

All this is very serious, and these problems should be treated by your vet. For acute infections, conventional therapy is to use antibiotics, and to combat dehydration with saline intravenous drips. Chronic cases may need similar treatment. Drugs may be given to control vomiting and convulsions. Often symptoms can be controlled by giving the dog a suitable diet. As I have said before, treatment of kidney disease does need to be controlled by your vet.

Homeopathy can be a very helpful in the battle to control nephritis. I recommend using:

Aconitum Napellus 6c in the very early stages of an acute infection. This helps to control the dog's fear and anxiety. It may also help to control the infection and limit damage to the kidneys. It is of most benefit if given before there is damage to the kidneys.

Apis Mellifica 30c helps to reduce the swelling which invariably occurs in acutely infected kidneys.

Arsenicum Album 30c for the dog who drinks little and often. It can also control vomiting and diarrhoea. Often, the coat is harsh and dry.

Belladonna 30c for acute infections where the dog may be hot and excited or when the pupils of the eyes are dilated. The urine may be a dark colour.

Berberis Vulgaris 30c when there is a great deal of pain over the back. The urine may be yellow.

Kali Chloricum 6c for the dog who dribbles copiously from the mouth. The dog may have ulcers in the mouth, or a greenish diarrhoea.

Lycopodium 30c when there is red sediment in the urine. It suits the thin dog who looks old, and may have a liver problem.

Mercurius Corrosivus 30c when urine is passed with a lot of painful straining. The urine may be bloodstained, or contain green pus. The dog is very thirsty, and there is a constant cycle of drinking and vomiting. In these cases water should be withheld until vomiting is under control, because your dog actually vomits more fluid than he drinks.

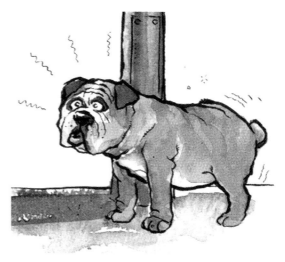

Ooh, that stings!

Natrum Muriaticum 6c when the dog is very thirsty, thin and losing weight.

Phosphorus 30c when vomiting occurs shortly after, but not immediately after, drinking water. Controlling vomiting can help to prevent dehydration and the need for intravenous drips. Phosphorus also acts as a tonic to the kidney tissues.

Plumbum Metallicum 6c when there is weakness or paralysis of the hind legs. The area of the lumbar spine may appear thin because the muscles have wasted away.

Silicea 30c to reduce the scar tissue in chronically damaged kidneys. It is particularly helpful to the dog who has always been thin.

Thuja Occidentalis 6c when there is pain over the kidneys, and pain in passing urine.

Urtica Urens 3x to help the flow of urine and the removal of poisonous waste products.

Explanation of Terms
Nephrosis is the name used to describe degeneration and death of the kidney tissue. Usually it is caused by chemical poisons. The poisonous products from severe burns and badly infected wounds also can cause the problem.

Pyelonephritis is an infection of the lower part of the kidney, where the urine collects before it passes to the bladder. This infection usually comes from an infection of the bladder passing upwards to the kidney.

The symptoms of both these conditions can be treated with the same remedies as nephritis.

Bladder

Cystitis is the name given to an inflammation of the bladder. It may be caused by an infection which has come up from the urethra, the tube through which urine is passed. Any blockage or paralysis which prevents urine being passed may create conditions in which infections can flourish. Conventional treatment for these infections is with antibiotics.

Cystitis may also be caused by the presence of 'stones' in the bladder. These stones develop from substances which come out of the urine as sediment. This may be helped by bacterial infection, or by a hereditary defect.

In the bitch very large stones may be found in the bladder. In male dogs small stones from the bladder frequently pass into the urethra, causing an obstruction. In both cases the dogs make frequent straining movements to pass urine but can pass only little or no urine. Where stones are actually present, there is no doubt that the conventional treatment of removing the stone surgically is essential. This does not prevent further stones from occurring, so the stones are analysed and the dog is put on a suitable diet or treated with suitable drugs to prevent further stones from forming.

Homeopathy can be used to relieve the painful symptoms, and to help prevent further infections, or further stones being formed.

Berberis Vulgaris 6c as a constitutional remedy where the liver may not function normally. The urine may be red, and the lumbar region of the back may be tender.

Cantharis 6c for the dog who strains violently. He can only pass a few drops of blood-stained urine.

Causticum 30c for chronic, recurrent cystitis. It is particularly useful in the older dog. It also helps when cystitis is caused by the bladder being over-distended. There may have been an obstruction or paralysis of the bladder.

Hydrangea 3x to prevent the formation of further stones. The urine may contain sediment which looks like white sand. These small white grains can grow as further material comes out from the urine, and form larger stones.

Lycopodium 30c as a constitutional remedy, where the liver may not be functioning normally. The dog may be thin, and look old. Small stones are formed and the urine may be red.

Nux Vomica 6c when an obstruction has been caused by post-operative paralysis of the bladder.

Urtica Urens 3x to increase urine flow, and decrease the likelihood of stones being formed.

Incontinence

This is most common in the older dog, and I have discussed the remedies in the section on the older dog (see page 69).

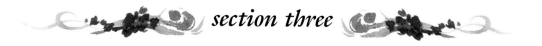

the remedies

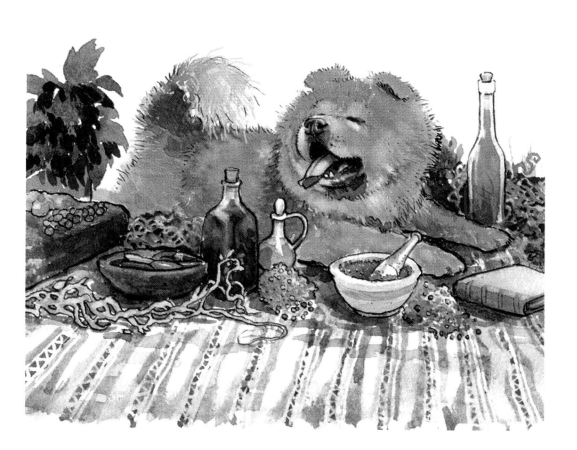

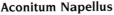

Aconitum Napellus

Aconitum napellus is made from Monkshood (*Aconitum napellus*), a wild plant found on heaths and commons. It is useful in the early stages of infections, for shock and for fear. Therefore it is indicated for the fearful, anxious character. Symptoms are made worse when the dog is indoors and at night. Its use is discussed in the sections on behaviour, the back, bones, coughs, diarrhoea, ears, eyes, first aid, the mouth, the nervous system, the nose, the male dog and urinary system problems.

Aethusa Cynapium

Aethusa cynapium is made from the wild plant Fool's Parsley, or Lesser Hemlock (*Aethusa cynapium*). It suits the anxious, whimpering dog, and is used in some cases of diarrhoea and for the skin. Symptoms are worse when the dog is warm, in the summer and indoors. Its use is discussed in the sections on pregnancy and skin problems.

Agaricus Muscarius

Agaricus muscarius is prepared from fresh toadstools. In dogs, it is mainly used for treating problems of the nervous system. It suits the fearless, indifferent dog. Symptoms are worse when the dog is in open, cold air, and before a thunderstorm. Its use is discussed in the sections on the nervous system and skin problems.

Agnus Castus

Agnus castus is made from the ripe berries of the Chaste Tree or Abraham's Balm (*Vitex Agnus castus*). The tree is found on the shores of the Mediterranean Sea. As its name implies, to eat the berries in quantity makes people chaste! It is mainly used in dogs to treat lack of sexual drive. It suits the introspective dog, lacking in courage. Its use is discussed in the section about male dog problems, and the section on pregnancy.

Alumina

Alumina is made from the chemical compound aluminium oxide. In dogs, it is used as a remedy to help weakness in old age. Symptoms are worse for the dog being in a warm room. Its use is discussed in the sections on the older dog, the skin and constipation problems.

Aconitum Napellus (monkshood) can be found growing in rocks in mountainous areas. It can be recognised by the helmet-like shape at the top of each flower.

Ammonium Carbonate

Ammonium carbonate is made from the chemical compound of that name, commonly called Sal Volatile, or smelling salts. It suits the overweight dog who dislikes exercise. Symptoms are worse in cold, wet weather. It is useful in dogs for treating lung and skin problems. Its use is discussed in the sections on coughs, the older dog and skin problems.

Apis Mellifica

Apis mellifica is made from honey bee venom. As you would expect from a bee sting, it is useful for swellings and puffiness, particularly when the swelling is tight with fluid. It helps the dog who prefers to be outside. Symptoms are worse in heat, and when the area is touched or pressed. Its use is discussed in the sections on backs, eyes, the female dog, first aid, joints, the mouth, pregnancy, the skin and tummy problems.

Argentum Nitricum

Argentum mitricum is made from silver nitrate. It suits the older, fearful and trembling dog. It is used to treat inflammations of mucous membranes. Symptoms are made worse by warmth. Its use is discussed in the sections on behaviour, eyes, the older dog and urinary system problems.

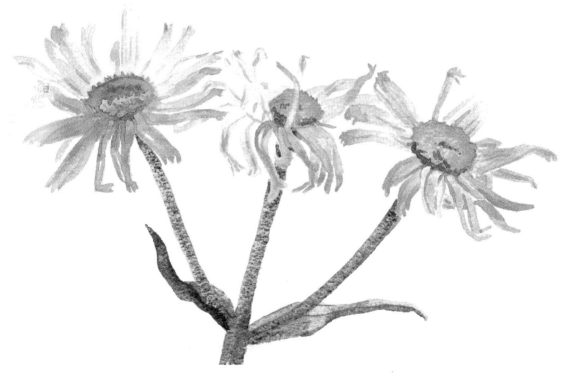

Arnica Montana (Leopard's Bane)
This yellow-flowered plant grows in the mountains. Its flower is very untidy and ragged, and looks somewhat like a poor relation to the dandelion.

Arnica Montana

Arnica montana is made from Leopards Bane or Mountain Tobacco. This plant comes from Central Europe and has untidy, golden, daisy-like flowers. The remedy is used for injuries where there is bruising or pain. It also reduces shock. It can be given before surgery to reduce both shock and bruising. It is indicated for the dog who is afraid of being touched or approached. Also, it suits the indifferent, morose dog. Symptoms are made worse by damp and cold, and by the area being touched. Its use is discussed in the sections on behaviour, the back, bones, ears, first aid, joints and the mouth.

Arsenicum Album

Arsenicum album is made from the chemical compound Arsenic Trioxide. It is used to treat all the extensive symptoms associated with arsenic poisoning. The dog may be restless, particularly at night. It suits the leaner and fearful dog. Symptoms are worse when the dog is cold and during wet weather. Its use is discussed in the sections on diarrhoea, ears, the nose, the older dog, pregnancy, the skin, tummy problems and the urinary system.

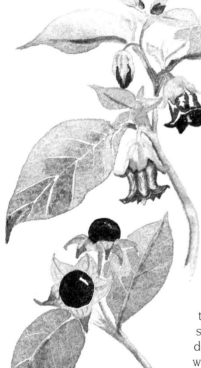

Astacus Fluviatilis

Astacus fluviatilis is made from the freshwater crayfish, or crawfish (*Astacus fluviatilis*). Its use in dogs is confined to treating skin rashes which cover the whole body. Symptoms may be worse when the dog is in the open air.

Asterias Rubens

Asterias rubens is made from the common starfish (*Asterias rubens*). It is used in dogs for treating tumours of the breast gland. It suits the flabby, overweight dog. Its use is discussed in the sections about the female dog and tumours.

Belladonna 30c

Belladonna is made from the well-known, poisonous wild plant, Deadly Nightshade. It acts on every part of the nervous system. It is used for treating excitement, aggression, hot and burning sensations, and for convulsions. The pupils of the dog's eyes are often dilated. Symptoms are made worse by the dog being touched or lying down, by noise, draught and and during the afternoon. Its use is discussed in the sections about behaviour, coughs, ears, pregnancy problems, first aid, male dog problems, the mouth, the nervous system and urinary system problems.

Belladonna (Deadly Nightshade) Every part of this plant is highly poisonous, not just the berries which are so attractive to children.

Berberis Vulgaris

Berberis Vulgaris is made from the roots of Barberry, a spiny shrub found in hedges and copses. It is useful when there are liver, kidney or bladder problems. It suits the heavy dog who has little stamina. It also helps painful conditions involving nerves. Symptoms are worse when the dog moves. Its use is discussed in the sections about the back, tummy problems and the urinary system.

Borax

Borax is made from the chemical compound Sodium Borate. It is helpful in treating irritating lesions which may discharge. It is particularly helpful in treating inturning eyelids (entropion) and mouth ulcers. Your dog may be frightened by sudden noises, such as gunshots and thunder. It is very helpful to the dog who is afraid of downward movement. Symptoms are worse in warm weather. Its use is discussed in the sections about behaviour, eyes, diarrhoea and mouth problems.

Bryonia Alba

Bryonia Alba is made from the climbing wild flower, White Bryony, and is suitable for the irritable dog who likes to stray. Symptoms are made worse by warmth, movement and eating, and made worse in the morning. It is useful for treating problems where mucous membranes are dry. Examples are coughs, and arthritic joints which are worse for movement. Its use is discussed in the sections about behaviour, the back, constipation, diarrhoea, the female dog, first aid, joints, the nervous system and older dogs.

Cactus Grandiflorus

Cactus Grandiflorus is made from the tropical American cactus, the Night Blooming Cereus. It is suitable for sad, ill-humoured or anxious dogs. Its main use in dogs to is to treat diseases of the heart valves.

Bryonia Alba (White Bryony) The whole plant is very poisonous. A few berries from this attractive plant can kill a child.

101

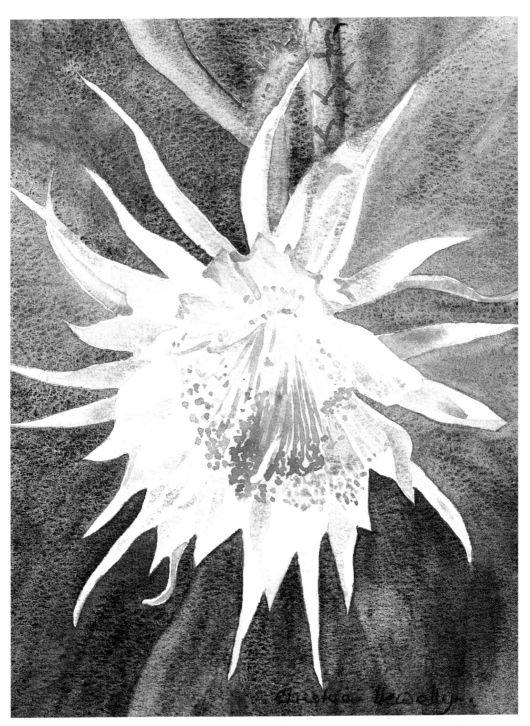

Cactus Grandiflorus (Night Blooming Cereus) is a tropical American cactus with very attractive flowers.

Calcarea Carbonica
Calcarea Carbonica is made from pure calcium carbonate, from oyster shells. It is of great benefit to the fat, sluggish and fearful dog. It is of particular help to the young dog with problems of bone growth and teeth. Symptoms may become worse during exertion, cold and wet. Its use is discussed in the sections about behaviour, the back, bones, constipation, eyes, female problems, the nose, puppies, skin problems and tumours.

Calcarea Fluorica
Calcarea Fluorica is made from the chemical compound calcium fluoride, sometimes called Fluorspar. It is found in bones, where it helps harden the bone structure. It is very useful in treating hard lumps in tissues. Symptoms are worse after rest. Its use is discussed in the sections on anal problems, bones, eyes, female problems, joints, the mouth, the skin and tumours.

Calcarea Phosphorica 30c
Calcarea Phosphoricum is made from the chemical compound calcium phosphate. It is of great benefit to the leaner and more restless dog, and especially puppies. It is useful for problems with bones and teeth. Symptoms are worse for cold and wet. Its use is discussed in the sections about behaviour, bones, female problems and puppies.

Cantharis
Cantharis is made from the insect Spanish Fly, *Cantharides versicatoria*. It suits the noisy dog who becomes excited and furious. Its main use is for treating inflammations of the urinary and sexual organs. Symptoms are worse when the dog is approached or touched. Its use is discussed in the sections about the female dog, first aid, the skin and urinary system problems.

Carbo Vegetabilis
Carbo Vegetabilis comes from charcoal made from plants. It suits the fat, lazy dog. It helps conditions where there is not enough oxygen in the blood. The dog's skin or gums may appear blue. It may also help the dog who does not appear to have fully recovered from an illness. Symptoms are worse in the evening and at night, for cold and open air, and in warm damp weather. Its use is discussed in the sections about constipation, coughs, diarrhoea, first aid, tummy problems and older dogs.

Carcinosin
Carcinosin is prepared from cancerous epithelial tissue. It is used in the treatment of cancers of epithelial tissues. Epithelial tissue is the lining tissue found in all organs and glands, for example, it includes the lining of the mouth, mammary glands and the skin.

Caulophyllum
Caulophyllum is made from the root of the North American plant Blue Cohosh (*Caulophyllum thalictroides*). This is a female remedy and is particularly useful for the whelping bitch. It can also lessen pain and stiffness in the small joints of the knees, ankles and toes. Its use is discussed in the sections about the female dog, joints and pregnancy.

103

Causticum

Causticum is made from the chemical compound Caustic Potash. It is useful in treating the more chronic problems, especially in older dogs. It has a particular action on arthritic, rheumatic and paralytic conditions. Symptoms are worse for cold dry weather and cold winds. Its use is discussed in the sections about the back, coughs, ears, joints, pregnancy, the nervous system, the older dog and urinary system.

Chamomilla

Chamomilla is made from the plant German Chamomile (*Matricaria chamomilla*). It suits the restless, sensitive and irritable dog, and is especially helpful to young dogs and puppies. Symptoms are worse for heat, fresh air, and in high winds. Its use is discussed in the sections on behaviour, diarrhoea, the mouth, male dogs, the nervous system, puppies and skin.

Chamomilla (German Camomile) is anti-inflammatory, and is traditionally used in Camiomile Lotion.

Cina Maritima

Cina Maritima is made from the unopened flower heads of the plant Wormseed (*Cina maritima*). It is a remedy for treating young dogs that are irritable, have an inconsistent appetite and may have fits (seizures). Symptoms are worse at night, in the sun and in summer. Its use is discussed in the sections about diarrhoea, the nervous system and puppy problems.

Cinchona Officinalis

Cinchona Officinalis is made from the bark of the Peruvian Cinchona tree, which contains quinine. The common name for this tree, and the remedy, is China and comes from the Peruvian word for quinine, Quina or Kina. The remedy is of particular help after debilitating illnesses. It is indicated for the dog who is indifferent, sulky and disobedient. Symptoms may be worse when the dog is touched and at night. Its use is discussed in the sections on behaviour, coughs, diarrhoea, the nose and puppies.

Cocculus

Cocculus is made from the berries of the Indian Cockle (*Anamirta cocculus*). This is a native climbing plant of the Malabar district of India and of Sri Lanka. In England, in the past, sometimes the berries were used to strengthen the intoxicating power of beer. The remedy is especially suitable for bitches with light coloured coats. It is used in dogs to

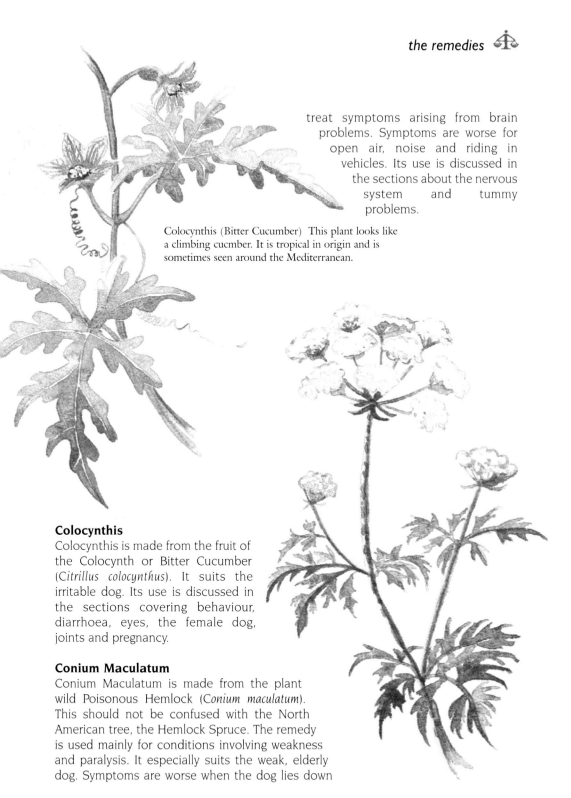

treat symptoms arising from brain problems. Symptoms are worse for open air, noise and riding in vehicles. Its use is discussed in the sections about the nervous system and tummy problems.

Colocynthis (Bitter Cucumber) This plant looks like a climbing cucmber. It is tropical in origin and is sometimes seen around the Mediterranean.

Colocynthis
Colocynthis is made from the fruit of the Colocynth or Bitter Cucumber (*Citrillus colocynthus*). It suits the irritable dog. Its use is discussed in the sections covering behaviour, diarrhoea, eyes, the female dog, joints and pregnancy.

Conium Maculatum
Conium Maculatum is made from the plant wild Poisonous Hemlock (*Conium maculatum*). This should not be confused with the North American tree, the Hemlock Spruce. The remedy is used mainly for conditions involving weakness and paralysis. It especially suits the weak, elderly dog. Symptoms are worse when the dog lies down

Conium Maculatum(Hemlock) In the year 399 BC, the Greek philospher Socrates was found guilty of heresy and sentenced to death. He drank a ccup of hemlock, which was the poison used for judicial executions in Ancient Greece. Sheakespeare's witches in *Macbeth* used hemlock in their brew.

105

and turns. Its use is discussed in the sections on eyes, female problems, the male dog, the nervous system, the older dog, skin problems and tumours.

Convallaria Majalis

Convallaria Majalis is made from the Lily of the Valley. Although grown as a garden plant, the Lily of the Valley is a common wild plant, found in most of Europe. The remedy is used in dogs to treat irregular heart beats. Its use is discussed in the section on the older dog.

Convallaria Majalis (Lily of the Valley) regulates the heart. The 16th century herbalist, John Gerard, said, "it strengthens the brain, and renovates a weak memory"!

Diesel Smoke

Diesel Smoke is made from – smelly diesel smoke! It is used for dogs who are sensitive to the smell and helps to control travel sickness. Its use is discussed in the section on tummy problems.

Drosera

Drosera is made from the wild plant Sundew. This plant is found on wet moors and in peat bogs. It is used for problems of the respiratory system, especially for prolonged spasms of coughing. Symptoms are worse at night and after resting. Its use is discussed in the section on coughs and the nervous system.

Euphrasia

Euphrasia is made from the wild plant Eyebright. It has a specific action on inflammations of the eye where hot painful tears are present. Symptoms are worse in the evening, indoors and when the dog is warm. Its use is discussed in the section on eye problems.

Ferrum Picricum

Ferrum Picricum is made from the chemical compound Iron Picrate. It suits dogs with dark coats. The remedy's main use is for treating enlarged prostate glands but is also helpful in painful infections of the urinary system and for treating warts. Its use is discussed in the sections on the male dog and tumours.

Euphrasia (Eyebright) is a 'bright-eyed' flower, which is used in eye lotions.

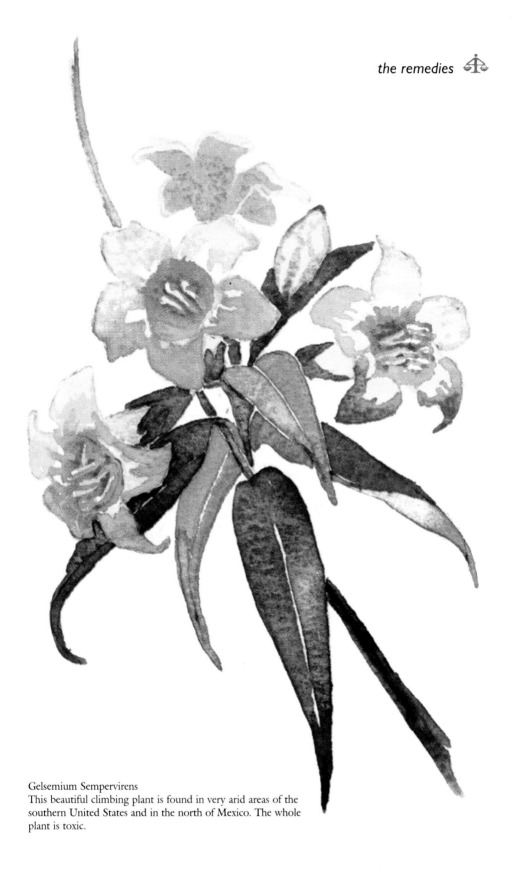

Gelsemium Sempervirens
This beautiful climbing plant is found in very arid areas of the
southern United States and in the north of Mexico. The whole
plant is toxic.

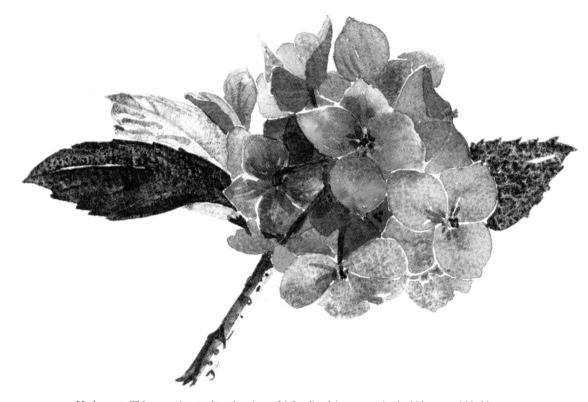

Hydrangea This attractive garden plant is useful for dissolving stones in the kidneys and bladder.

Gelsemium Sempervirens 30c
Gelsemium Sempervirens (see picture on page 107) is Yellow Jasmine, also called Carolina Jasmine and False Jasmine. It is useful for treating nervous symptoms, especially those associated with muscular weakness and paralysis, and fear and trembling. Symptoms are worse in damp weather and before a thunderstorm. Its use is discussed in the sections covering behaviour, diarrhoea, first aid, joints, the nervous system and the older dog.

Graphites
Graphites is made from Black Lead, the form of carbon used in pencil lead. It suits the dog who is overweight, has a cold skin, and a tendency to be constipated. It is also used to treat skin problems. Symptoms are worse for warmth and at night. Its use is discussed in the sections on constipation, ears, eyes and skin.

Hamamelis Virginica
Hamamelis Virginica is made from the bark of the shrub Witch Hazel. It has a particular action on problems of bruising and blood blisters. Symptoms are worse for warmth and moist air. Its use is discussed in the section on ears.

Hekla Lava
Hekla Lava is made from volcanic ash. It is used to treat lumps and tumours on bones. It may also be used when parts of the bone have died. It is particularly useful for bones

of the face and upper jaw. Its use is discussed in the sections covering the back, bones and mouth problems.

Hepar Sulphuris Calcareum

Hepar Sulphuris Calcareum is made from the chemical compound Calcium Sulphide. It suits the lightcoated, sluggish and sensitive dog. The remedy is used for treating painful infections, especially when there is pus. Symptoms are worse for dry, cold winds and draughts. Its use is discussed in the sections on bones, coughs, ears, first aid, male dogs, the mouth, the nose, the female dog and skin.

Hydrangea

Hydrangea is made from the leaves and young shoots of the garden shrub *Hydrangea arborescens*. It is used in dogs to prevent stones forming in the urinary bladder, and to treat enlargement of the prostate gland. Its use is discussed in the sections about the male dog and the urinary system.

Hydrastis Canadensis

Hydrastis is made from the root of the North American plant Golden Seal (*Hydrastis canadensis*). This remedy suits the older, easily tired dog. It is used for thick, ropy and yellow discharges. Its use is discussed in the sections on ears, the female dog, the male dog, the nose and tumours.

Hyoscamus Niger (Henbane)
In 1910, Dr Crippen used hyoscine, a poison from this plant, to murder his wife. Every part of the plant is poisonous. Animals will not go near it because of its smell.

Hyoscyamus Niger

Hyoscyamus Niger is made from Henbane, which is found mainly in the southern half of England, in sandy soils and near the sea. The pale flowers have many dark, purple veins. It is useful for treating the excited, hysterical dog who may like to fight. It helps the suspicious, jealous dog. Symptoms are worse at night and when the dog is lying down. See the sections on behaviour, coughs, diarrhoea and the older dog.

Hypericum Perforatum

Hypericum Perforatum is made from the wild plant St John's Wort. This is the perforate species, which is especially common on chalky soils. It is a remedy which is particularly useful for injuries to nerves. It is of great importance in treating wounds where nerve endings are damaged, and also in the treatment of puncture wounds. Symptoms are worse in cold and damp conditions. Its use is discussed in the sections about the back, first aid, joints and skin.

Ignatia

Ignatia is made from the seeds of the St Ignatius Bean (*Strychnos amara*). It suits the dog who may have changeable moods, both gentle and hysterical. The remedy is most useful in counteracting the effects of grief and worry. Therefore it is used when a dog is upset because it has been deprived of a companion, or has had a change of home. Symptoms may be worse in the morning and outdoors. Its use is discussed in the sections about behaviour, the nervous system, the older dog, pregnancy and puppy problems.

Ipecacuanha

Ipecacuanha is made from the root of the South American plant *Cephalis ipecacuanha*. It suits the dog who is irritable and intolerant. The remedy is used to treat nausea and vomiting, coughing and associated problems. Symptoms are worse for warm moist air and after the dog has rested. Its use is discussed in the sections on coughs, the nose and tummy problems.

Kali Arsenicum

Kali Arsenicum is made from the chemical compound known as Fowlers Solution, a combination of Arsenious Acid and Potassium Carbonate. Its use for dogs is discussed in the section on skin problems.

Kali Chloricum

Kali Chloricum is made from the chemical compound Potassium Chlorate. Its main use is in treating problems of the urinary system. Its use is discussed in the sections on the mouth, the older dog and the urinary system.

Lachesis

Lachesis is made from the venom of the Bushmaster Snake. It is helpful in treating haemorrhages, Septicaemia and the collapsed dog. Also, it is indicated for the suspicious, jealous character. Symptoms are worse after sleep. Its use is discussed in the sections covering behaviour, the female dog, first aid, the nose and pregnancy.

Ledum Palustre

Ledum palustre is made from the plant Marsh Tea (*Ledum palustre*). This is a native plant of bogs in Scotland. It suits the dog whose body, or whose wounds, feel cold. This is a very useful remedy for treating puncture wounds and insect bites. Symptoms are worse when the dog is warm and at night. Its use is discussed in the sections on coughs, eyes, first aid, joints, the older dog, skin problems and tumours.

Lycopodium

Lycopodium is made from the crushed spores of Club Moss. It has a strong action on digestive, liver and kidney disorders. It suits the dog with a mild temperament, who is afraid of being alone and also suits the dog who is thin. Symptoms are worse for heat. See the sections about behaviour, constipation, the male dog, the older dog, the skin, tummy problems and the urinary system.

Mercurius Corrosivus

This is made from the chemical compound Mercuric Chloride. It is used to treat the symptoms associated with chronic kidney disease. Symptoms are worse in the evening and at night. Its use is discussed in the sections on diarrhoea, ears, eyes, the male dog, the mouth, tummy problems and the urinary system.

Mercurius Solubilis

Mercurius Solubilis is made from the metal Mercury. It is useful in conditions where tissues are degenerating. Symptoms are worse at night and in a warm room. They are also worse in damp or wet weather. The remedy is discussed in the sections on diarrhoea, eyes, the male dog, the mouth, the nose and the skin.

Mezereum

Mezereum is made from the bark of the flowering shrub Spurge Olive (*Daphne mezereum*). It suits the dog who is very sensitive to cold air. Symptoms are worse for cold air, at night, and when the dog is touched or active. Its use is discussed in the section on skin problems.

Natrum Muriaticum

Natrum Muriaticum is made from common salt, Sodium Chloride. It is useful in treating the thin, thirsty dog. It suits the dog who is irritable and does not like to be consoled. Symptoms are worse for noise and heat. Its use is discussed in the sections on eyes, the nervous system, the older dog, skin problems and the urinary system.

Hypericum Perforatum (Perforate St John's Wort) In mediaeval times, it was thought to drive away devils and evil spirits, so it was hung in doorways and windows.

Nitricum Acidum

Acidum Nitricum is made from Nitric Acid. It is used for symptoms you would expect to see from contact with acids. It is particularly useful for lesions where the skin joins the linings of body orifices, or body openings, such as the lips and nostrils. It suits the irritable dog who is sensitive to noise, or to being touched. Symptoms are worse at night. Its use is discussed in the sections on anal problems, constipation, the eye, the male dog, the mouth and the nose.

Nux Vomica

Nux Vomica is made from the poison Strychnine which comes from the seeds of the Poison Nut, *Strychnos Nux-vomica*. Conventional medicine has used strychnine, even though it is poisonous, in small doses as a stimulant and tonic for hundreds of years. It is suitable for the dog who is thin, nervous and irritable with a fiery temperament. It is very helpful for tummy problems. Symptoms are worse in the morning, for dry weather and cold. Its use is discussed in the sections on the back, behaviour, constipation, the nervous system, tummy problems and the urinary system.

Mezereum (Daphne Mezereum) The whole plant, including the bark, is very poisonous. It is essential to keep children away from it, which is difficult as it is very pretty.

Petroleum

Petroleum is made from Petroleum Oil or Crude Rock Oil. It suits the dog who is irritable and easily upset. The remedy is used in dogs for treating problems of the skin and for travel sickness. Symptoms are worse when the dog is cold and damp, and in thunderstorms. Its use is discussed in the sections on the skin and tummy problems.

Phosphoricum Acidum

Phosphoricum Acicum is made from Phosphoric Acid. It is used to treat the debilitated or 'run down' dog. It helps both physical and mental problems, and is particularly useful in the young dog. It suits the dog who appears listless and indifferent. Symptoms are worse when the dog is cold or has exerted itself. Its use is discussed in the sections on behaviour, bones, the male dog, puppies and tummy problems.

Nox Vomica (Poison Nut) contains strychnine. Dr Morell treated Hitler with a medicine containing strychnine. It is thought that Hitler's abuse of this drug caused his terrifying temper.

112

Phosphorus

Phosphorus 30c is made from the substance Phosphorus. It is used for problems when degenerative and destructive changes are taking place, such as in chronic kidney disease. As so many diseases cause tissues to be destroyed, Phosphorus is useful for a wide variety of problems in dogs. It suits the fearful dog who is thin and always hungry. Symptoms are worse when the dog is touched, after exertion and during thunder storms. Its use is discussed in the sections about the back, behaviour, coughs, eyes, female problems, first aid, male problems, the mouth, the nose, older dogs, tummy problems, tumours and the urinary system.

Phytolacca

Phytolacca is made from the plant Poke Root or Virginian Poke (*Phytolacca decandra*). It suits the indifferent dog. In dogs, the remedy is used for glandular swellings, mainly the mammary glands. Symptoms are worse when the dog is wet, during cold wet weather, and for movement. Its use is discussed in the sections on the female dog, the mouth, pregnancy, puppies and tumours.

Picricum Acidum

Picricum Acidum is made from the chemical compound Picric Acid (Trinitrophenol). In dogs its main use is for treating excessive sexual excitement, and enlargement of the prostate gland. Symptoms are worse for wet weather, hot weather and exertion. Its use is discussed in the sections on behaviour, eyes and the male dog.

Plumbum Metallicum

Plumbum Metallicum is made from the metal Lead. It is used to treat painful conditions which lead to paralysis. For example, a painful slipped disc in the back can lead to paralysis of the hind legs. Its use is discussed in the sections on the back, the nervous system and urinary system.

Psorinum

Psorinum is made from the dried skin blisters caused by mange mites. It suits the smelly dog who is sensitive to cold. The remedy is used for problems where there are offensive discharges, especially skin problems. Symptoms are worse in hot sunshine. Its use is discussed in the sections on ears and skin.

Pulex Irritans

Pulex Irritans is made from the common flea, *Pulex irritans*. It is used to treat dogs who are allergic to fleas. Giving one tablet once a week, when fleas are active, may prevent the allergy. The remedy is discussed in the section on skin problems.

Pulsatilla

Pulsatilla is made from the Windflower (*Anemone nemorosa*). It suits the gentle dog who has a yielding disposition and is particularly useful in treating bitches. The dog's behaviour may be changeable and contradictory. It prefers the open air. Symptoms are worse for heat, and in the evening. Its use is discussed in the sections on behaviour, diarrhoea, ears, eyes, the female dog, the male dog, the nose, older dogs, pregnancy and the skin.

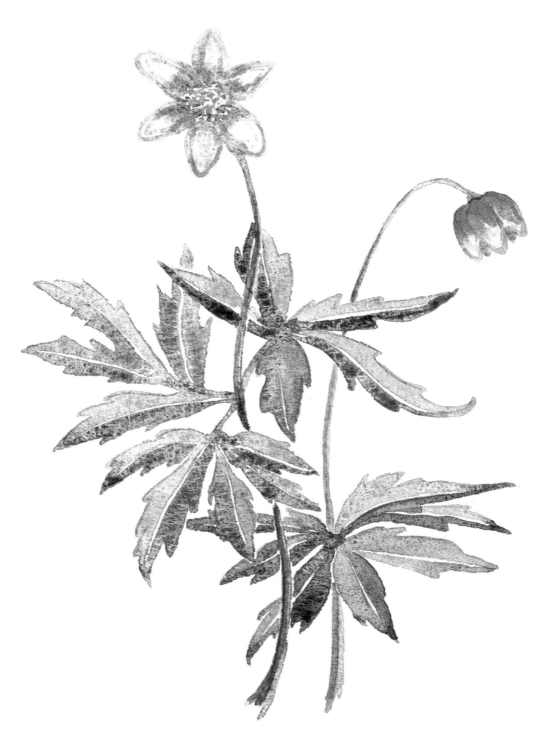

Pulsatilla (Wood Anemone or Windflower) gets its name because the flowers open in the wind and sun.

Rhus Toxicodendron

Rhus Toxicodendron is made from the North American plant, Poison Ivy. Contact with this plant is notorious for producing severe blisters of the skin and swollen joints, so the remedy is used for treating these kinds of problems. It suits the dog who is restless. Symptoms are worse when resting and at night, and for cold and wet weather. Its use is discussed in the sections on diarrhoea, the eye, joints, the mouth, the nervous system, the nose and skin problems.

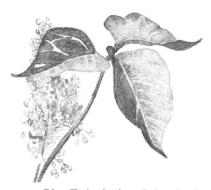

Rhus Toxicodendron (Poison Ivy) is found only in North American forests. Contact with this plant, even through clothes, causes a burning irritation which can last for weeks.

Ruta Graveolens

Ruta Graveolens is prepared from the shrub Common Rue. It is grown for decoration and as a medicinal herb. It is indicated for treating eye, tendon and joint problems. It is especially useful for injuries to the periosteum, the membrane which lines the surface of bones, and which produces new bone when bones are healing. Symptoms may be worse for resting and in cold wet weather. Its use is discussed in the sections on the back, joints and the nose.

Sepia

Sepia is made from the ink of the Cuttlefish. It is particularly suited to the bitch who is indifferent to family and puppies, irritable and easily offended. Symptoms are worse for cold air, in the evenings and during thunderstorms. Its use is discussed in the sections on behaviour, constipation, the female dog, older dogs, pregnancy and the skin.

Silicea

Silicea is pure flint. It is very useful in chronic conditions. It suits the dog that is anxious, sensitive and feels the cold. The remedy promotes the reabsorption of scar tissue and clears up chronic abscesses and pussy discharges. Symptoms are worse in the morning, and for damp or cold. Its use is discussed in the sections on bones, constipation, the eye, the nose, the skin and urinary system.

Spongia Tosta

Spongia Tosta is made from roasted Sponge. It is used to treat respiratory and heart problems, especially those aggravated by exertion, and anxiety. Symptoms are worse when the dog is going uphill or upstairs, and in high winds. Its use is discussed in the sections on coughs and the older dog.

Staphysagria

Staphysagria is made from the seeds of Stavesacre, or Wild Raisin (*Delphinium staphsyagria*). This plant is found in Southern Europe and Asia. It is used to treat symptoms where there is marked irritation, such as cystitis. It suits the dog which is sensitive but resents correction. Symptoms are worse when the dog is angry and for cold. Its use is discussed in the sections on behaviour, eyes and skin problems.

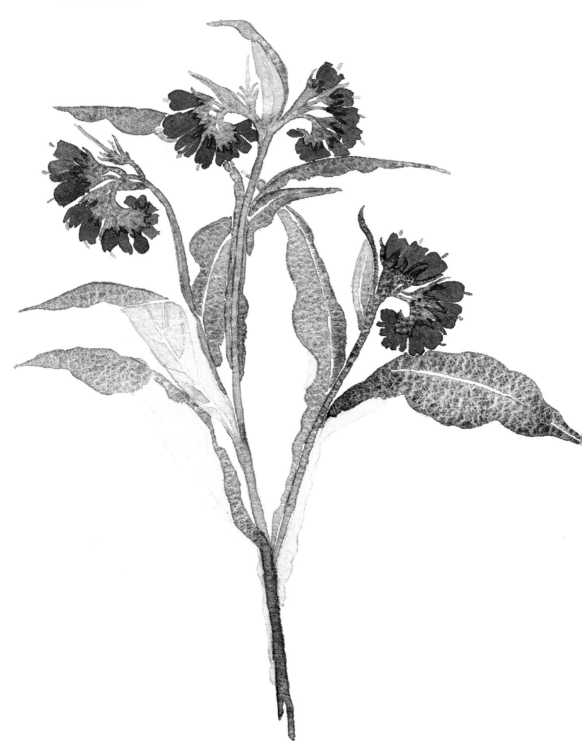

Symphytum (Common Comfrey, Boneset or Knitbone)
The old names describe the plant's properties in helping bones to heal.

Sulphur

Sulphur is made from the element sulphur, which is well known as a cure for many irritable skin complaints. The remedy suits the smelly dog, with a harsh dry coat, that dislikes water. It can enhance the action of other remedies. Symptoms are worse for resting and heat. Its use is discussed in the sections about constipation, ears, the nose and the skin.

Symphytum

Symphytum is made from the herb Comfrey or Knitbone (*Symphytum officianale*), which is commonly found near rivers and canals. As the plant's name implies, it is a great remedy for encouraging bones to heal. Its use is discussed in the sections about bones and the eye.

Tarentula Hispania

Tarentula Hispania is made from the Spanish Spider, a wolf-spider from southern Europe. It is used to treat the hysterical and restless, destructive and oversexed dog. Moods alter suddenly. Symptoms are worse when the dog moves or is being touched, and noise. Its use is discussed in the sections about behaviour, the female dog, the male dog and the nervous system.

Tellurium

Tellurium is made from the metal Tellurium. It is very useful for chronic skin problems. Symptoms are worse at night, during cold weather, and when scratching or rubbing. Its use is discussed in the sections on ears, eyes and skin problems.

Thallium

Thallium is made from the metal Thallium. It suits the dog who trembles and is weak on his hind legs. Its use is discussed in the sections on the older dog and skin problems.

Urtica Urens (Stinging Nettle) For centuries, man has both hated the stinging nettle and needed it. The stinging nettle has been used to make cloth, as food and in medicine.

117

Thuja Occidentalis

Thuja Occidentalis is made from the green leaves of the North American conifer Arbor Vitae (*Thuja occidentalis*). The remedy is used for treating warty growths and tumours. Its use is discussed in the sections about anal problems, the eye, the female dog, the nose, the skin, tumours, and urinary system problems.

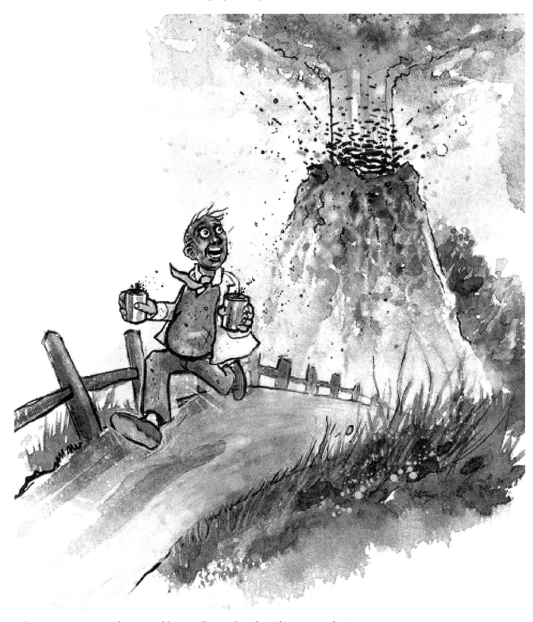

As you can see, many homeopathic remedies are based on dangerous substances ...

Urtica Urens

Urtica Urens is made from the common stinging nettle. Therefore it has an obvious use in treating painful, irritating rashes. The remedy is also useful in both promoting and discouraging milk flow. When it is in very high potency, it promotes milk production. In very low potencies it reduces the amount of milk. Its use is discussed in the sections on the eye, the female dog, first aid, pregnancy, puppies, the skin, and urinary system.

Ustilago Maydis

Ustillago Maydis is made from the Corn Smut, a fungus which turns the grains of corn into a black powder. Its use in dogs is discussed in the section about skin problems.

Zincum Metallicum

Zincum Metallicum is made from the metal Zinc. This remedy is useful for chronic conditions where tissues appear to wear out faster than they are repaired. It suits the dog who is very sensitive to noise, is tired and may appear stupid. Symptoms may appear worse in the early evening. Its use is discussed in the sections on eyes, the male dog, the nose, the nervous system and pregnancy.

The Nosodes

The nosodes are homeopathic remedies made from the part of the body which is diseased. For example, canine parvovirus nosode is made from infected diarrhoea and blood taken from a dog with the disease. The infected material is diluted in the homeopathic way to produce potencies similar to ordinary homeopathic remedies.

Using the principle of treating like with like, nosodes can be used to treat specific diseases. Also, they can help a dog who has not been well since having a disease. He may have recovered from a disease but it has left a problem. For example, a dog who has recovered from parvovirus may still have problems with frequent diarrhoea.

I have not discussed the uses of nosodes in this book because they treat a disease, not the symptoms you can see. So, to use nosodes properly, you need to have an accurate diagnosis of the dog's disease problem. This can only be done satisfactorily by your vet. Treating diseases with nosodes does require the help of a vet who uses homeopathy.

However, there two nosodes which you can use. These are Carcinosin, which is made from cancerous epithelial tissue, and Pulex Irritans, which is made from fleas. These nosodes are discussed in the sections on tumours and the skin.

Also, nosodes can be used to prevent disease. They can be used as the homeopathic equivalent of a vaccine. This is discussed in the section on Puppy Problems (page 77).

Conclusion

As you can see, many homeopathic remedies are based on dangerous substances. Dr Hahnemann took a great risk all those years ago, but has given us a method of treating illnesses which is now used all over the world and with a great degree of success. We don't know who first thought of using lava to treat bone problems or Diesel Smoke to help prevent travel sickness, but there is no doubt that more remedies will be investigated and become available in the years to come.

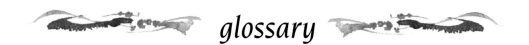

Acute Moist Eczema is an acute painful, raw and sore skin lesion. It can occur very suddenly, and on any part of the body. The lesion exudes clear fluid, which makes the hair matt over the lesion. Clipping the hair away from the lesion prevents it from spreading.

Allergen is the substance to which your dog may be allergic. For example, if your dog is allergic to fleas, then the flea is the allergen.

Anal Adenoma is a tumour of glandular tissue around the anus.

Aural haematoma is a blood blister in the ear flap. The ear flap becomes filled with blood from a broken blood vessel.

Axillary lymph node is the lymph node in the dog's armpit.

Blepharitis is inflammation of the eyelids.

Callus is the bony swelling formed at the site of a fracture when the bone is healing.

Cataract is an opacity of the lens of the eye. It appears as a greying of the pupil of the eye. Eventually the pupil becomes completely white and opaque, causing blindness.

Chalazion is a painless swelling on the border of the eyelid. It is not infected.

Chorea is the term used for persistent involuntary twitching of muscles.

Conjunctiva is the membrane lining the inside of the eyelids.

Conjunctivitis is inflammation of the membrane lining the inside of the eyelids.

Constitutional Remedy is a homeopathic remedy which deals with the whole patient, not just the symptoms of the problem.

Cornea is the clear membrane in the front of the eyeball, through which light passes into the eye.

Cryosurgery is the surgical destruction of tissue by freezing it.

Cystitis is an inflammation of the urinary bladder. It may be caused by infection or by 'stones' forming in the bladder.

Diabetes Mellitus, or 'Sugar Diabetes', is a condition where sugar metabolism is faulty. Sugar accumulates in the blood, causing damage to the kidneys and other organs.

Dry Eye is a condition where the insufficient tears are produced in the eye. The cornea becomes dry, and is easily infected or damaged.

Ectropion is the term used for eyelids which droop, or turn outwards, exposing the conjunctiva.

Electroencephalogram is a tracing recording the electric currents in the brain. It is made by a special machine called an electroencephalograph.

Emphysema is a condition where the tissues lining the inside of the lung leak, and allow air to enter the supporting tissue of the lung. (Let us make an over-simple comparison. If you think of a lung as a sponge, the air is normally contained in the holes. In emphysema, the air has got into the structure of the sponge.) The lung becomes less efficient and loses its elasticity, making breathing difficult.

Entropion is the term used when the eyelids turn in, and the margins of the lids and eyelashes rub on the surface of the cornea.

Epithelium or *Epithelial Tissue* is the layer of cells lining mucous membranes in animals. It is continuous with the skin. For example, the epethelium lining the mouth is continuous with the skin of the lips.

Epulis is a hard tumour, or growth, on the gums.

Exostosis is an abnormal bony lump on a bone.

Glaucoma is a condition where the pressure inside the eye becomes excessive. The eye is painful and may become swollen. Eventually, the internal structure of the eye is destroyed by the pressure, causing blindness.

Granuloma is a tumour which appears as a prominent mass of sore tissue.

Hip Dysplasia is an hereditary condition where the hip joint is not correctly formed.

Homeopathic potency is the strength of a homeopathic medicine. It is expressed as the number of dilutions the remedy has undergone. For example, a remedy that has been diluted one hundredfold, six times, has a potency of 6c.

Inguineal lymph node is the lymph node situated in the groin.

Jaundice is the condition where the dog's tissues turn yellow as a result of liver disease. The yellow colour is seen easily in the whites of the eyes and the gums.

Keratocoele is the name given to the swelling on the surface of the cornea which is caused by the eye contents protruding through a perforated cornea.

Lipoma is a tumour of fat cells. It usually appears as a soft swelling beneath the skin and is not cancerous.

Lymph nodes or 'glands' are the structures through which fluid drains from the body.

Each gland has its own territory, and filters out invading organisms, such as bacteria and cancerous cells. Probably we are most familiar with the 'glands' in our armpits and groins.

Mammary tumour is a tumour in a mammary or breast gland.

Mastitis is an infection of a mammary or breast gland.

Molar teeth are the crushing teeth at the back of a dog's mouth. They are also called cheek teeth.

Mucous Membrane is the lining of internal organs, and is covered with mucus. It consists of a layer lining the surface, the epithelium, and a supporting layer containing glands, blood vessels and nerves.

Nephritis is the name given to an inflammation of the kidney. Usually it is caused by an infection.

Nephrosis is the name given to the destruction of the kidney tissue by a poison. This may be a substance such as Phosphorus, or a poison produced by bacteria.

Nosode is a homeopathic remedy produced from an infecting organism, or from infected tissues or discharges.

Osteomyelitis is an infection of bones.

Osteoporosis is the condition where the mineral content of the bone decreases, and the bones become brittle.

Periorbital eczema is an inflammation of the skin around the eyes. The eyelids and skin may thicken, or be sore and discharging.

Polyp is a tumour which projects outwards, often with a narrow neck or stalk.

Potency: see Homeopathic potency.

Premolar teeth are the three or four teeth between the canine and molar teeth in each jaw.

Progressive Retinal Atrophy is an inherited disease of dogs, in which the retina progressively wastes away, leading to blindness.

Proving is giving a substance, or a remedy, in doses so large that the symptoms which one is trying to cure are aggravated.
Pulmonary oedema is the condition where static fluid collects in the lungs.

Pyometra is a condition found only in bitches, where fluid and pus collect in the womb.

Ranula is a blocked and swollen salivary gland duct. It appears as a large blister in the mouth, usually under the tongue.

Retina is the light-sensitive membrane at the back of the eye.

Retinal Atrophy is a wasting away of the retina, leading to blindness.

Sebaceous cyst is a blocked and swollen sebaceous gland.

Sebaceous gland is a gland in the skin which produces sebum.

Sebum is the substance which keeps the skin moist and supple.

Sinusitis is an infection of the sinuses in the head, around the nose.

Spay is to remove the ovaries and womb of a bitch.

Staphyloma is a swelling of the damaged part of a cornea, Pressure from within the eye causes the cornea to bulge.

Stye is a painful swelling on the margin of the eyelid.

Urethra is the tube through which urine passes during urination.

Uveitis is an inflammation of all the structures within the eyeball.

Vesicle is a swelling like a blister, filled with fluid. Vesicles may single or multiple, and may be large or small.

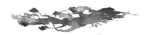 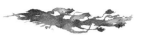 # *useful addresses*

British Association of Homoeopathic Veterinary Surgeons
Hon. Secretary: Mr C E I Day, MA, Vet.MB, MRCVS
Alternative Medicine Centre
Stanford-in-the-Vale
Faringdon
Oxfordshire SN7 8NQ

The British Veterinary Association
7 Mansfield Street
London W1M OAT

Ainsworths Homeopathic Pharmacy
36 New Cavendish Street
London W1M 7LH

Video
A 60-minute video with Geoffrey Llewellyn is available from APV Films, 6 Alexandra Square, Chipping Norton, Oxon OX7 5HL (01608 641798). Geoffrey works with a variety of dogs to cover all aspects of dog ownership, from buying a puppy to caring for a dog in old age.

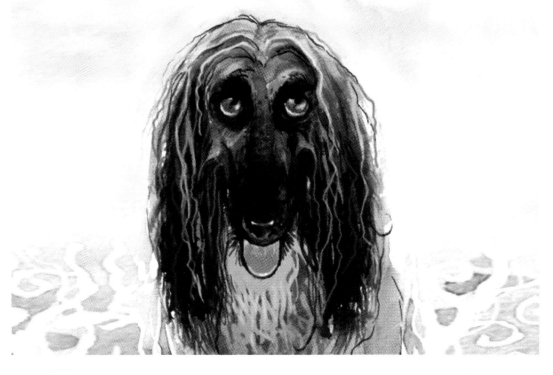

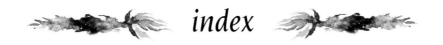

index